A Seminar on Antigen-Antibody Reactions Revisited

A Seminar on Antigen-Antibody Reactions Revisited

Editor

Carol A. Bell, MD
Department of Pathology
Brotman Medical Center
Culver City, California

Presented at the

35th Annual Meeting of the
American Association of Blood Banks
Anaheim, California
1982

Mention of specific commercial products or equipment by contributors to this American Association of Blood Banks publication does not represent an endorsement of such products by the American Association of Blood Banks, nor does it necessarily indicate a preference for those products over other similar competitive products.

Efforts are made to have publications of the AABB consistent in regard to acceptable practices. However, as new developments in the practice and technology of blood banking occur, AABB's Committee on Standards recommends changes when indicated from available information. It is not possible to revise each publication at the time each change is adopted. Thus, it is essential that the most recent edition of the *Standards for Blood Banks and Transfusion Services* be used as the ultimate reference in regard to current acceptable practices.

American Association of Blood Banks
National Office
1117 North 19th Street, Suite 600
Arlington, Virginia 22209

Edited by Carol A. Bell, MD
Director of Publications: Rosanne Sheehan

ISBN No. 0-914404-80-6
First Printing
Printed in the United States of America

Committee on Annual Meeting Seminar

Carol A. Bell, MD, Chairman
George Garratty, FIMLS, MRC Path, Vice-Chairman

Marilyn K. Moulds, MT(ASCP)SBB
Paul Ness, MD
Susan Moore Steane, MT(ASCP)SBB
M. Jane Wilson, MT(ASCP)SBB

The Emily Cooley Lecturer

Today's lecture is the twentieth in a series of annual lectures in honor of Emily Cooley, an outstanding medical technologist.

Emily Cooley was an attractive young woman reared in a distinguished family—her grandfather had been a Justice of the Supreme Court of Michigan and her father was a professor of pediatrics at Wayne State University. She had been brought up to be an artist, or a writer, or simply to preside over a household like her mother. She had attended a private school for girls and graduated from Vassar with a degree in landscaping. Her mother, a kindly, gracious woman, was often incapacitated with attacks of melancholia and her father, then about to retire, was ailing much of the time. Emily ran the household and was her father's companion, chauffeur, traveling aide, nurse, secretary and illustrator. It was she who drew the beautiful illustrations of blood films that appeared in Dr. Cooley's publications.

After the death of both of her parents, Emily had to find a career in which to earn a living. Having been so intimately connected with medicine, and hematology in particular, she chose medical technology. She took her training at Henry Ford Hospital and received a Master's Degree before she started work. Returning to Children's Hospital, where her father had worked in the laboratory, she became the chief hematology technician. An excellent morphologist, Emily became the mainstay of her department and was looked up to and beloved by her colleagues.

Emily Cooley was not only a fine technologist and a dedicated worker in the laboratory but she was a warm, sensitive, intelligent and gracious human being. It is to her memory that this series of lectures is dedicated.

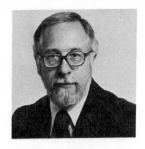

The 1982 Emily Cooley Memorial Lecturer Edwin A. Steane, PhD

Dr. Edwin A. Steane was trained in medical technology in Birmingham, England, and was certified by the Institute of Medical Laboratory Sciences. Emigrating to Canada in 1957, he was chief technologist at Plummer Memorial Hospital in Sault Ste. Marie, Ontario, before becoming a research technologist at Milwaukee Blood Center in 1961. He received a BS in chemistry with honors from the University of Wisconsin and a PhD in physiology from George Washington University in 1973, with minors in biochemistry and immunology. He served as Technical Director of the National Red Cross Blood Program from 1973-1976. Born in Coventry, England, he became an American citizen in 1965 and a "naturalized" Texan in 1976. Dr. Steane is currently Associate Professor of Clinical Pathology in the Department of Pathology, Southwestern Medical School, at the University of Texas Health Science Center at Dallas, and is Associate Director of the Blood Bank at Parkland Memorial Hospital.

His research interests have been in molecular mechanisms in biology, particularly antigen-antibody interaction and membrane structure and function. Author and coauthor of over 20 papers and numerous abstracts dealing with soluble metabolites in red cells, red cell metabolism, and red cell membrane effects, Dr. Steane has written chapters in several books on the physical chemistry of hemagglutination and interaction of antibodies with red cell surface antigens. He has participated in numerous AABB Workshops, served as Chairman of the Scientific Section Coordinating Committee and is currently Treasurer of the AABB.

An American jazz afficionado, and past president of the International Association of Jazz Record Collectors, he has participated in album production for the Smithsonian Institute, edited and published *Jazz Digest*, a magazine of jazz record reviewers, and is part owner of the jazz record company, Phoenix Jazz Records, which has more than twenty (20) LPs on the market. He lives with his wife Susan Moore Steane in Dallas.

Participating in AABB's 1975 Preconvention Seminar, Dr. Steane's subject was "The physical chemistry of agglutination." In this seminar, as an Emily Cooley Lecturer, he carries us several steps further.

Emily Cooley Lecturers

1963 .... E. Eric Muirhead, MD
1964 .... Scott N. Swisher, MD
1965 .... Wolf W. Zuelzer, MD
1966 .... Alexander S. Wiener, MD
1967 .... M. M. Strumia, MD
1968 .... Hugh Chaplin, Jr., MD
1969 .... Emanuel Hackel, PhD
1970 .... Flemming Kissmeyer-Nielsen, MD, PhD
1971 .... Neva Martin Abelson, MD
1972 .... Bernard Pirofsky, MD
1973 .... Serafeim P. Masouredis, MD
1974 .... Paul J. Schmidt, MD
1975 .... Eloise R. Giblett, MD
1976 .... Richard E. Rosenfield, MD
1977 .... Herbert F. Polesky, MD
1978 .... Mary N. Crawford, MD
1979 .... Professor Sir John Dacie, MD
1980 .... Kathryn M. Beattie, MT(ASCP)SBB
1981 .... Prof. Dr. C. P. Engelfriet

Contents

1   Red Cell Membrane and Antigen Topography **1**

Blood Group Antigens and Membrane Structure 1
Fluid Mosaic Model 6
Antigenic Determinants 7
References 12

**2   Monoclonal Antibodies: A New Tool to Probe the
Biologic Membrane** **15**

Introduction 15
Polyclonal vs. Monoclonal Antibodies 15
Monoclonal Antibodies to Detect the Presence
   of Virus 17
Monoclonal Antibodies Against Parasites 18
Monoclonal Antibodies Against Tumor
   Differentiation Antigens in Man 19
Monoclonal Antibodies to the Major
   Histocompatibility Complex in Man 20
Summary 20
References 21

**3   Nonisotopic Immunoassays in Blood Group
Serology** **23**

Introduction 23
The Evolution of Immunoassays 24
Type of Immunoassays 25
Practical Aspects 34
Application to Blood Group Serology 39
Conclusion 41
Appendix: Reaction Equations 42
References 43

**4   Antibody Uptake: The First Stage of the
Hemagglutination Reaction** **47**

Introduction 47
Definitions 48

Physicochemical Basis of Antigen-Antibody Binding . 50
Effect of Environmental Factors on Antigen-Antibody
  Reactions 58
Summary 63
References 64

5   The Emily Cooley Lecture—Red Blood Cell
     Agglutination: A Current Perspective 67

Introduction 67
A Brief Historical Note 68
General Concepts 71
The Second Stage of Agglutination 76
Concluding Remarks 92
References 94

6   Potentiators of Agglutination 99

Introduction 99
"Complete" and "Incomplete" Antibodies 101
Potentiation by Human Serum or Plasma 102
Bovine Albumin and Other Viscous Solutions as
  Potentiators of Agglutination 103
Developments in the Practical Use of Potentiators 113
Enhancement of the Indirect Antiglobulin Reaction . . 124
Summation and Conclusion 126
References 127

7   Action and Application of Enzymes in
     Immunohematology 133

Introduction 133
Serologic Uses of Enzymes 139
Applications of Enzymes 162
Conclusion 163
References 164

8   Elution of Antibody from Red Cells 175

Introduction 175
Historical Review 175
The Mechanisms of Elution 177

Factors That Influence the Outcome of Elution
    Techniques 182
Elution Studies in the Evaluation of Blood Samples
    with a Positive DAT 188
Applications of Adsorption-Elution Tests 194
Further Applications of Elution 196
Considerations in the Selection of Elution Methods .. 200
Appendix 1:   Cold Acid Elution 210
Appendix 2:   Lui Easy-Freeze Elution 211
Appendix 3:   Xylene Elution 211
Appendix 4:   Chloroform Elution 212
Appendix 5:   Elution by Sonication 213
Appendix 6:   Chloroquine Dissociation of IgG 213
References 214

9   **The Use of Antigen-Antibody Techniques in
Forensic Serology** **223**

Introduction 223
The Typical Problem 224
The Principles of Inhibition, Mixed Agglutination
    and Elution as Applied to the Detection of
    Antigens in Blood Stains 226
The Detection of HLA Antigens in Blood Stains 236
Summary 236
Appendix: A Microelution Technique for the
             Detection of Red Cell Antigens in
             Blood Stains 237
References 238

Index **241**

Introduction

In recent years, these seminars have dissected antigens (1980), and immune destruction of cells by both alloantibodies (1981), and auto-antibodies (1979). These presentations themselves have been a reprise of problems encountered in compatibility testing (1972). Yet it is still possible to add to our knowledge of the reaction that is the basis for immunohematology, a revisit to the antigen-antibody reaction itself. In this review, we explore the laboratory techniques developed in the past 10 years which allow new ways to demonstrate the old reaction. These new methods include the use of nonisotopic techniques and of monoclonal antibodies. The membrane model in the latter is not a red cell, but a virus. These membrane probes have been used to explore the red cell membrane topography itself and, in turn, knowledge of membrane morphology and chemistry has allowed us to manipulate the technology further. This seminar also addresses the phases of the antigen-antibody combination and the forces involved, forces which we have used empirically over the years without knowing how or why they worked. With this information as background, we can discuss the ways in which we can manipulate the reaction by potentiating agglu-tination, altering the red cell membrane enzymatically, and inter-preting antigen and antibody by absorption and elution. Finally, we discuss one of the ultimate applications of the antigen-antibody reac-tion, forensic serology. We know you will find this revisit informative and helpful in using the reaction in new and imaginative ways your-selves and for the benefit of your patients and science.

Carol A. Bell, MD
Editor

1
Red Cell Membrane and Antigen Topography

Serafeim P. Masouredis, MD, PhD

T HE ANTIGEN IN ANTIGEN-ANTIBODY REACTIONS can be either on a hapten or macromolecule in solution, which commonly results in precipitation of the immune complex, or on a particulate or cellular component. When the reaction involves a blood group antigenic determinant on the red blood cell it may result in diverse phenomena, ranging from complement fixation and hemolysis to complex cellular interactions involving immunoprotein coated red cells and macrophages. The classical and by far the most clinically useful reaction is the occurrence of hemagglutination.

Different aspects of the antigen antibody reaction will be addressed by the other authors in this book. This introductory presentation will provide a summary of our current understanding of red cell blood group antigens from the perspective of membrane structure.

Blood Group Antigens and Membrane Structure

Blood groups are antigenic determinants on the red cell membrane. Their accessibility to antibody for crosslinking to produce agglutination indicates that they are surface-oriented antigenic components on the membrane.

Over a period of some 80 years in excess of 400 antigenic specificities distributed over more than a dozen blood group systems have been identified using the relatively simple and unsophisticated technique of immune hemagglutination. Although there is a wealth of information on the serology of blood group antigens, there has been, until recently, little or no knowledge concerning the molecular nature of these antigens and their relationship to the red cell membrane.

Serafeim P. Masouredis, MD, PhD, Professor of Pathology, Director, University Hospital Blood Bank, University of California, San Diego, School of Medicine, La Jolla, California

The red cell membrane for obvious reasons is one of the most extensively studied biological membranes. They are readily obtainable and membranes can be prepared easily by controlled hypotonic lysis. It may be hazardous, however, to use them as a general model since red cells are highly specialized with respect to their unique mechanoelastic properties. Deformability of red cells is a very specialized property which appears to be required for the continuous and repeated stresses of transversing through small diameter capillaries for a period of time in excess of 100 days.

RBC Membrane Ultrastructure

The RBC shape and morphology at the microscopic level is well known. Electron microscopy of fixed sections provides little information other than the RBC membrane is uniform and is about 90 A wide.

The technique of freeze-fracture and etching is more revealing. In this method red cells frozen at −150 C are fractured in liquid nitrogen by cutting with the microtome. The freeze-fracturing process hemisects the lipid bilayer, splitting the bilayer to expose two complementary surfaces facing the cleavage plane. A platinum-carbon replica made of the fracture faces can then be examined by transmission electron microscopy. When this is done particles about 85 A diameter are found on the fracture faces which are called intramembranous particles (IMP).[1] These particles are asymmetrically distributed on the two fracture surfaces, there being more on the protoplasmic face as compared to the extracellular face.

The human red cell has about 1/2 million of these IMP. They are puzzling structures and a great deal of effort has gone into determining their composition and function. Using a variety of techniques, IM particles can be shown to consist of at least two membrane proteins, glycophorin A (PAS-1), and component 3.[2] A particularly striking property of the particles is their ability to undergo redistribution and aggregation under a variety of environmental changes, such as temperature changes, a decrease in pH or ionic strength, protease modification of the red cell, and following ligand binding to surface receptors.[3]

The freeze-fracture techniques may be helpful in determining the blood group antigen-bearing component. Water adjacent to the membranes may be sublimed away with heat which results in deep-etching and exposes the external surface of the membrane. If the antigen-bearing component is represented in the intramembranous particle, then binding of a ferritin-labeled antibody to the surface of the red cell could result in redistribution of the particles that would correspond with the distribution of the ferritin on the surface of the cell.

An additional technique for studying the ultrastructural features of the membrane is the use of immunoferritin conjugates to label antigenic determinants on the membrane. This technique has the potential for both revealing the distribution pattern of the antigen and for estimating their numbers. Results obtained with this technique will be presented below.

Chemical Composition RBC Membrane

The gross chemical structure of the red cell membrane is not too informative except to indicate that red cell membranes are similar in their protein and lipid composition to other biological membranes (about 50% protein and 50% lipid).

RBC Membrane Proteins

A more informative analysis of membrane proteins can be obtained through the use of sodium dodecyl sulfate-polyacrylamide gel electrophoresis (SDS-PAGE). Briefly, membranes are solubilized in the ionic detergent, SDS, so that the proteins are dissociated and denatured. They are then subjected to electrophoresis in an SDS-containing polyacrylamide gel. Under these conditions, the membrane polypeptides migrate in the gel according to their molecular weights. The polypeptides can be identified in the gel by staining for protein (Coomassie blue) or for carbohydrate with the periodic acid Schiff (PAS) stain.[4]

There are a large number of bands in the protein stained gel, each corresponding to a polypeptide. The molecular weights range from 240,000 at the top of the gel to 29,000 at the bottom. By using special techniques, the method is capable of identifying 20-30 polypeptides. Only about eight to ten major polypeptides are readily identified with the usual method. There are at least four distinct sialoglycoproteins, two of which form complexes that give rise to three additional bands in the PAS-stained gel.

Table 1 summarizes the properties of the membrane polypeptides identified on SDS-PAGE. It shows the molecular weights, the percentage of the total for each polypeptide, the number per cell and their membrane location. Although SDS-PAGE is a powerful technique, it is important to emphasize that it does not provide any information concerning the architecture of the membrane, the relationship of these polypeptides to each other, or their functional arrangement in the membrane.

Membrane proteins have been classified on the basis of operational criteria into two types: peripheral and integral. Peripheral proteins are

Table 1.—Major Red Blood Cell Membrane Proteins

Band	Mol. Weight	Name	Location*	Percent Total	No. Copies/Cell
1	240,000	Spectrin	P	25	200,000
2	220,000	"			
2.1	200,000	Ankyrin	P	5	100,000
2.2	190,000				
2.3	180,000				
3	93,000	Anion exch.	I	25	1,000,000
4.1	78,000		P	4-5	200,000
4.2	72,000		P	4-5	200,000
5	43,000	Actin	P	4-5	400,000
6	35,000	G3PD**	P	4-5	500,000
7	29,000		P	4-5	500,000
8	23,000		P	1	150,000
PAS Bands					
PAS-2	31,000	Glycop. A	I	1-2	400,000
PAS-3	24,000	Glycop. B	I	0.5	100,000
PAS-1	(dimer PAS-2)				

* P = peripheral, I = integral
**Glyceraldehyde-3-PO_4 dehydrogenase

weakly bound to the membrane and can be dissociated and solubilized by relatively mild conditions, such as, high ionic strength solutions, metal chelating agents, etc. Peripheral proteins usually go into solution free of membrane lipids and are soluble and molecularly dispersed in neutral aqueous buffers; so that in many respects they resemble soluble proteins. Integral proteins, in contrast, require for solubilization hydrophobic bond-breaking agents such as detergents, organic solvents, or chaotropic agents. When solubilized they are usually associated with lipids and are insoluble or aggregated in aqueous buffers.[5]

In addition to categorizing the SDS-PAGE polypeptides as either peripheral or integral proteins, it is possible to determine the membrane location of each major red cell polypeptide (Table 1) using a variety of different techniques. Only band 3 and the PAS-staining sialoglycoproteins are found on the external surface of the membrane. These polypeptides and any other polypeptides present in too low a concentration to stain with Coomassie blue or PAS are the prime candidates for either protein or glycoprotein blood group antigens. All

4

of the peripheral proteins are found on the cytoplasmic face of the membrane and most of these polypeptides make up the cytoskeleton of the red cell. They contribute about 60% of the membrane protein and form a complex two-dimensional network at the cytoplasmic surface of the membrane which serves to maintain cell shape and deformability.[6]

The cytoskeleton may be of no immediate interest with respect to blood group antigenic activity. Although there is no experimental evidence, the cytoskeleton may participate indirectly in surface phenomena involving antigenic receptors by restricting or facilitating their mobility. Such would be the case if the Rh antigens are on band 3 which is linked to the cytoskeleton. Component 3 is a major transmembrane polypeptide which contains a small amount of carbohydrate and constitutes almost 25% of the total membrane protein. It is involved in anion transport and probably other processes.

As reviewed below, all the external glycopeptides have been associated with blood group antigenic activity.

RBC Membrane Lipids

Lipids constitute about 50% of the weight of the RBC membrane. Two classes of lipids, phospholipids and cholesterol, make up the bulk of the lipids both occurring in about equal molar amounts so that the cholesterol to phospholipid molar ratio under normal conditions is about 0.95. Glycolipids occur in small amounts (about 1%) and in addition to glycoproteins carry carbohydrate determinants for ABH, Ii and P blood groups.

The phospholipids make up the lipid bilayer backbone of the membrane. They are amphiphilic in having two domains, a strongly hydrophilic head group consisting of phosphate and its linked moiety and a hydrophobic portion due to one or two fatty acid chains. In aqueous solutions phospholipids will spontaneously form bilayers. The phospholipids (just as the membrane proteins) are asymmetrically distributed. The polar groups of phosphatidylcholine and sphingomyelin are predominantly on the outer surface, whereas phosphotidylethanolamine and phosphotidylserine are on the inner surface.

Red cell lipids, in addition to carrying blood group determinants, indirectly influence the activity of these antigens. Rh antigen activity is lipid dependent,[7] and the cholesterol content of the membrane may indirectly affect the expression of some antigens. Cholesterol is noncovalently inserted into the lipid bilayer and the quantity of cholesterol can be either decreased or increased. Alterations in the cholesterol content affects the bilayer fluidity. Such changes may affect mobility of membrane components or by other poorly defined mechanisms the expression of blood group antigens as discussed below.

Fluid Mosaic Model

A productive model of membrane structure has been the fluid mosaic model of Singer and Nicolson.[8] Briefly, it postulates that the membrane consists of a lipid bilayer some 70-90 A thick (as shown by EM) which forms a continuous two-dimensional lipid phase. The lipids are arranged in a bilayer so that the hydrophobic acyl chains point toward the center of the bilayer and hydrophilic heads (phosphate groups, etc.) are arranged on either side of the bilayer facing the aqueous environment.

Inserted into the bilayer are proteins, some of which penetrate the bilayer completely (transmembrane) and others only partially on the cytoplasmic aspect of the bilayer. Hydrophobic amino acids are found in the penetrating segments of the protein (as has been shown for glycophorin A),[9] which allows the protein to interact with the hydrophobic interior of the bilayer.

An important feature of the model is that both lipids and proteins are asymmetrically distributed on either side of the membrane, as indicated previously. There is an additional concept proposed in the fluid-mosaic model, which is that both lipids and protein can undergo, under appropriate influences, lateral diffusion in the plane of the membrane, as demonstrated above with the aggregation of IMP. The rate of motion of proteins is much slower, probably 100-fold slower than membrane lipids. In addition, there are protein-protein interactions as well as lipid-lipid and protein-lipid interactions, as indicated, for example, by the reversible loss of Rh antigen activity following lipid removal.[7]

Both mobility and specific interactions of membrane components are believed to be related to the functional activity of membranes. These concepts may have implications for blood group antigens. If the membrane component (lipid or protein) contains a receptor, such as a blood group antigen, then mobility or clustering of the receptor bearing component, may influence or modulate the function of the receptor. Phenomena such as immune hemagglutination, macrophage interaction and so forth may be significantly affected by component mobility and aggregation.

6

Antigenic Determinants

Table 2 lists some of the types of information that would be useful in associating blood group antigenic determinants with membrane structure.

Table 2.—Membrane Aspects of Blood Group
Antigenic Determinants

---

1. Number per red blood cell
2. Orientation and two-dimensional distribution
3. Chemical and/or conformational structure of the determinant
4. Identification of membrane bearing component
5. Association with other membrane elements and membrane organization
6. Biological function

Number Determinants Per Cell

The number of accessible determinants would be expected to play an important role in serological phenomena and other types of blood group antigen-antibody interactions. Although with some antigens, as in the case of D,[10] the quantity of antigen per red cell may be constant, there is evidence that with other blood group antigens there may be significant variability in antigen content from cell to cell, as has been reported for A.[11] Furthermore, the methods used to measure the number of determinants on intact cells only provide preliminary data, which can only be confirmed when the specific membrane component bearing the antigen is identified.

A variety of methods have been used to determine the number of immunologically accessible blood group antigens per cell. The qualification accessible implies that it may be possible that there are more determinants in the membrane than are available on the unmodified native membrane. Commonly used methods include: (1) radiolabeled antibodies, either primary, or secondary (anti-IgG)[12]; (2) labeled staphylococcal protein A; (3) immunoelectron microscopy[13-16]; and (4) enzymatic release for carbohydrate antigens as determined from the quantity of immunodominant sugar removed by a glycosidase. Of all these methods, immunoelectron microscopy has the potential of providing both the spatial distribution of determinants on the surface of the membrane, and an estimate of their numbers.

Table 3 shows previously published values for the red cell Rh antigen sites as determined with the use of radiolabeled antibodies[12]

Table 3.—Blood Group Antigen Sites Per Red Blood Cell

Antigen	Probable Genotype	Site Number Per Cell	Method
Rh			
c	$R_2 R_2$	35,000	Imm. conj.
	cc	85,000	I* anti-IgG
	cC	53,000	I* anti-IgG
C	$R_1 R_1$	31,000	Imm. conj.
E	$R_2 R_2$	30,000	Imm. conj.
	E	25,600	I* anti-IgG
e	$R_1 R_1$	22,000	Imm. conj.
	ee	24,400	I* anti-IgG
	eE	14,500	I* anti-IgG
D	$R_2 R_2$	30,000	Imm. conj.
	D+ cells	35,000	I* anti-IgG
ABH			
A_1		850,000	I* anti-A
A_2		240,000	I* anti-A
A_3		30,000	I* anti-A
B		2,200,000 (?)	Galactosidase
H	O	300,000	Imm. conj.
	B	200,000	Imm. conj.
	A_1	150,000	Imm. conj.
	A_1 B	100,000	Imm. conj.
	A_2 B	150,000	Imm. conj.
Duffy			
Fy^a	Fy(a+b−)	16,800	Imm. conj.
	Fy(a+b+)	7,500	Imm. conj.
Kidd			
Jk^a	Jk(a+b−)	14,400	Imm. conj.
Diego			
Di^b	Di(a−b+)	17,800	Imm. conj.
U	U+	23,300	Imm. conj.
Kell-Cellano			
k	kk	4,000	Imm. conj.
K	Kk	5,000	Imm. conj.
	KK	7,100	I* anti-IgG

Imm. conj. = immunoferritin electron microscopy[13-16]
I* = [^{125}I][12,16]
Site numbers are maximum values of range reported

8

and immunoelectron microscopy.[13] Values range from 10 to 85,000 sites per cell. The immunoconjugate values are in agreement with values obtained using radioisotopic techniques, except for the c and C antigens. Immunoferritin values for these antigens are about 1/2 of those found with isotopic techniques. The table lists saturation values for the data obtained by the radioisotopic method and equilibrium values for the immunoferritin technique. The immunoferritin values would be about 10-20% greater at complete saturation.

Table 3 also lists values for a number of other blood group antigens and the methods used to obtain the estimates. There is a wide variation in the number of antigens per cell, from 1-2 million for ABH to 3-7000 for Kell and Cellano antigens.

Distribution and Orientation

The topological distribution of blood group antigenic determinants on the surface is unclear. With ghost membranes using immunoelectron microscopy it appears to be random and aperiodic.[14] The use of ghost membranes in this technique, however, raises doubts that the ferritin patterns observed faithfully represent the antigen distribution on the native membrane.

Although the function of blood group antigens is unclear, they appear to be involved in recognition phenomena and would be expected to be found on the plasma side of the membrane. Membrane components, as discussed previously, are asymmetrically distributed and, in particular, all the membrane carbohydrate is on the outside ("sugar-coated"). As a result, blood group antigens with carbohydrate determinants would only be expected to be found on the outside surface of the membrane. Evidence has been presented, using ^{125}I-labeled antibodies and oriented vesicles, that the carbohydrate antigens, A and I, are found only on the outside surface of the membrane.[17]

A recent report[18] indicated that the D antigen is present on D-negative red cells but that it is found on the cytoplasmic side of the membrane. Because of the unusual nature of this report, the binding of labeled anti-D to right-side out and inside-out red cell vesicles from D-positive and D-negative red cells was tested. Methods are available for inverting RBC vesicles and acetylocholinesterase which is found only on the outside surface was used to assess the sidedness of the vesicle preparations. Table 4 summarizes the results. D antigen was present on only the external surface of D-positive red cells. No immunologically reactive D antigen was found on the inside of D-positive cells, nor on either the outside or inside of D-negative cells.[19]

Table 4.—IgG Anti-D Binding to Oriented Vesicles

| | Sidedness Assay | | | Anti-D Binding | |
| | Ach Activity* | | | | Relative |
Vesicle Preparation	Total	Surface Exposed	Percent Contamination	ng per μg protein	Binding as Percent
RO+	1.85	1.85	0	10.8	100
IO+	2.11	0.89	42	1.52†	14†
RO−	1.76	1.74	1	1.01	9.3
IO−	2.35	0.34	14	1.01	9.3

*Acetylcholinesterase (n mole/min/ug protein)
 Total obtained following TX-100 solubilization
†Values corrected for 42% sidedness contamination

Antigenic Determinant and Membrane-Bearing Component

The antigenic site of blood group antigens is defined by a specific conformation of a macromolecule containing either or both carbohydrate or amino acid residues. Most, if not all, current information on blood groups is with carbohydrate determinants based on the elegant studies of Kabat, Morgan, Watkins, Hakomori, and others. Carbohydrate determinants are found on oligosaccharide chains on glycosphingolipids or proteins. The carbohydrate chains are very heterogeneous with respect to their length and degree of branching, containing from 3 to 50 sugar residues.

Glycosphingolipids, a minor lipid component, carry carbohydrate determinants for ABH, Ii and P.[20] The oligosaccharides are attached to a ceramide moiety and the terminal sugars in the chain determine blood group specificity, N-acetyl galactosamine for A and galactose for B. The Ii antigens appear to reside in the middle of the chain. ABH and Ii antigens are also found on glycoproteins, bands 3 and 4.5.[21]

The MN antigens have been localized to the major sialoglycoprotein (PAS-2 or glycophorin A). The MN specificity is determined by heterogeneity in two amino acids at positions 1 and 5 from the amino terminus, serine-glycine for M and leucine-glutamic acid for N.[22] The Ss antigens have been associated with a minor sialoglycoprotein, PAS-3 or glycophorin B. A methionine-threonine polymorphism at position 29 appears to control the expression of S or s.[23]

There is general agreement that the Rh antigens are associated with a lipid-dependent membrane protein. There is considerable difference of opinion as to which membrane component carries the Rh antigens.

10

One group of investigators have associated the D antigen with a polypeptide of approximately 7000 daltons[24] and more recently they have produced evidence to indicate that the D antigen is on a proteolipid.[25] Another group has associated the D antigen with band 3[26] and a third group with a membrane protein of 28,500 daltons with additional components of 50,000 and 68,000 daltons.[27] This latter group also reported that Fy[a] is associated with 39,500 (possibly PAS-2), 64,000 and 88,000 dalton proteins. Table 5 summarizes some of the available information on antigen structure and membrane-bearing component.

Effect of Membrane Associations and Properties on Blood Group Antigen Activity

Perturbation of the lipid bilayer may play a role in altering blood group antigen accessibility to antibody. Cholesterol loading and de-

Table 5.—Structure of Antigenic Determinant and Membrane-Bearing Component

Blood Group Antigen	Structure Determinant	Antigen-Bearing Component
ABH	Carbohydrate	Glycosphingolipid Bands 3, 4.5
Ii	Carbohydrate	Glycosphingolipid Bands 3, 4.5
P	Carbohydrate	Glycosphingolipid
MN	Protein, a.a. polymorphism	PAS-1 and 2 (Glycophorin A)
Ss	Protein, a.a. polymorphism	PAS-3 (Glycophorin B)
Rh	? Protein ? Proteolipid	? Band 3 or ? 28-50,000 daltons membrane protein ? Polypeptide
Duffy	? Protein	? PAS-2 ? Band 3
Kell	?	?
Kidd	?	?

11

pletion of the membrane alters the reactivity of the D and A antigen. When red cells are loaded with cholesterol (C/PL = 1.55), the relative detectable number of D antigens per cell was about twice that observed with cholesterol depleted (C/PL = 0.65) red cells. In an analogous experiment, there was only a 20% increase in detectable A_1 antigen, suggesting that the A_1 antigen, in contrast to the D antigen, was in a more fully exposed position on the surface of the red cell membrane. This phenomenon may be important for other cell surface receptors, and has been described as passive modulation of blood group antigens.[28] These results have been confirmed using ^{125}I anti-D. Cholesterol depletion reduces anti-D binding, whereas cholesterol loading increases anti-D binding.[29,30]

Although remarkable progress has been made in unraveling the relationship between blood group antigens and membrane structure, there are still large gaps in our understanding of this fascinating subject. Until more information is available, it is to be expected that there will be considerable differences and controversy in the interpretation of the studies reported.

Acknowledgment

These studies were supported by National Institutes of Health grant HL12994.

References

1. Branton D. Fracture faces of frozen membranes. Proc Natl Acad Sci USA 1966;55:1048-56.
2. Pinto da Silva P, Nicolson GL. Freeze-etch localization of concanavalin A receptors to the membrane intercalated particles of human erythrocyte ghost membranes. Biochim Biophysica Acta 1974; 363:311-9.
3. Wise GE, Shienvold FL, Rubin RW. Effects of pronase and concanavalin A upon the freeze-etch morphology of cell membranes of intact human erythrocytes. J Cell Sci 1978;30:63-76.
4. Fairbanks, G, Steck TL, Wallach DFH. Electrophoretic analysis of the major polypeptides of the human erythrocyte membrane. Biochem 1971;10:2606-17.

5. Steck TL. The organization of proteins in the human red blood cell membrane. J Cell Biol 1974;62:1-19.
6. Lux SE. Dissecting the red cell membrane skeleton. Nature 1979;281:426-9.
7. Green FA. Phospholipid requirement for Rh antigenic activity. J Biol Chem 1968;243:5519-21.
8. Singer SJ, Nicolson GL. The fluid mosaic model of the structure of cell membranes. Science 1972;175:720-31.
9. Tomita M, Marchesi VT. Amino acid sequence and oligosaccharide attachment sites of human erythrocyte glycophorin. Proc Natl Acad Sci USA 1975;72:2964-8.
10. Rearden A, Masouredis SP. Autoradiographic estimation of red cell D antigen content using ^{125}I anti-D and ^{125}I membrane labeling. Blood 1977;50:971-9.
11. Reyes F, Gourdin MF, Lejone JL, Cartron JP, Gorius JB, Dreyfus B. The heterogeneity of erythrocyte antigen distribution in human normal phenotypes; an immunoelectron microscopy study. Br J Haematol 1976;34:613-21.
12. Huges-Jones NC, Gardner B, Lincoln PJ. Observations of the number of available c, D, and E antigen sites on red cells. Vox Sang 1971;21:210-6.
13. Masouredis SP, Sudora EJ, Mahan L, Victoria EJ. Antigen site densities and ultrastructural distribution patterns of red cell Rh antigens. Transfusion 1976;16:94-106.
14. Masouredis SP, Sudora EJ, Mahan L, Victoria EJ. Quantitative immunoferritin microscopy of Fy^a, Fy^b, Jk^a, U, and Di^b antigen site numbers on human red cells. Blood 1980;56:969-77.
15. Matsukura Y. Electron microscopic observations on the H antigen sites of human erythrocytes using ferritin antibody conjugates. Vox Sang 1976;31:321-31.
16. Cartron JP, Gerbal A, Hughes-Jones NC, Salmon C. 'Weak A' phenotypes. Relationship between red cell agglutinability and antigen site density. Immunology 1974;27:723-7.
17. Schenkel-Brunner H, Cartron JP, Doinel C. Localization of blood group A and I antigenic sites on inside-out and right-side-out human erythrocyte membrane vesicles. Immunology 1979;36:33-6.
18. Plapp FV, Evans JP, Tilzer LL. Detection of Rh_o(D) antigen on the inner surface of Rh negative erythrocyte membranes. Fed Proc 1981;40:208.
19. Kleeman JE, Masouredis SP, Victoria EJ. Exposure of the Rh_o(D) antigen on the surface and cytoplasmic domains of the red cell membrane. Immunology 1982;45:27-30.

20. Marcus DM, Kundu SK, Suzuki A. The P blood group system: Recent progress in immunochemistry and genetics. Semin Hematol 1981;18:63-71.
21. Hakomori S. Blood group ABH and Ii antigens of human erythrocytes: Chemistry, polymorphism, and their developmental change. Semin Hematol 1981;18:39-62.
22. Anstee DJ. The blood group MNSs-active sialoglycoproteins. Semin Hematol 1981;18:13-31.
23. Dahr W. Serology, genetics and chemistry of the MNSs blood group system. Blood Transfusion Immunohematol 1981;24:84-95.
24. Plapp FV, Kowalski MK, Tilzer L, Brown PH, Evans J, Chiga M. Partial purification of Rh_o (D) antigen from Rh positive and negative erythrocytes. Proc Natl Acad Sci USA 1979;76:2964-8.
25. Plapp FV, Brown PH, Sinor LT, Evans JP, Tilzer L. The Rh_o (D) antigen is a dicyclohexylcarbodiimide-binding protein. Transfusion 1981;21:601 (abstract).
26. Victoria EJ, Mahan LC, Masouredis SP. Anti-Rh_o (D) IgG binds to band 3 glycoprotein of the human erythrocyte membrane. Proc Natl Acad Sci 1981;78:2898-2902.
27. Moore S, Woodrow CF, McClelland DBL. Isolation of membrane components associated with human red cell antigens Rh(D), (c), (E) and Fy^a. Nature 1982;295:529-31.
28. Shinitzky M, Souroujon M. Passive modulation of blood group antigens. Proc Natl Acad Sci USA 1979;76:4438-40.
29. Basu MK, Flamm M, Schachter D, Bertles JF, Maniatis A. Effects of modulating erythrocyte membrane cholesterol on Rh_o (D) antigen expression. Biochem Biophys Res Comm 1980;95:887-93.
30. Victoria EJ, Masouredis SP. Unpublished observations.

2

Monoclonal Antibodies: A New Tool to Probe the Biologic Membrane

Paul E. Hurtubise, PhD

Introduction

IN 1975, KOHLER AND MILSTEIN,[1] with their observations concerning the molecular assembly of the immunoglobulin molecule, described a new method to "immortalize" a single antibody-producing cell line by fusion with mouse myeloma cells. This technology launched a new era in the development of more refined immunological probes to be used in the study of important antigenic structures associated with the biologic membrane. This hybridoma technology allows the generation of large amounts of homogeneous or monoclonal antibody that can be made available to basic investigators and clinical researchers to identify, isolate and characterize membrane structures that are important in our understanding of infectious processes, tumor development, cell maturation and differentiation, and the genetic control of membrane structures. These monoclonal antibodies are powerful serological and potentially therapeutic tools that can be used in the identification and control of disease. This chapter is a brief overview of the use of monoclonal antibodies in a few areas of biological investigation of membrane structures.

Polyclonal vs. Monoclonal Antibodies

The antibody response of an animal to a given antigen is highly complex. The type and magnitude of this response is under genetic control of the animal and is dictated by cell-to-cell interactions, complexity of the antigen, and the foreignness of the immunizing material to the animal. When all of these complex factors are brought together in an appropriate manner, the animal usually produces antibody that can be detected in the serum. The serum of the immunized animal contains a large number of antibodies directed to a large number of surface structures on the antigen. These various surface structures are

Paul E. Hurtubise, PhD, Department of Pathology and Laboratory Medicine, University of Cincinnati Medical Center, Cincinnati, Ohio.

called antigenic determinants. Some of these determinants are major and initiate the largest quantity of antibody. Some are minor and more subtle and produce minimal amounts of antibody. Collectively, the response is referred to as a polyclonal response to antigen with a multiplicity of various antibodies directed to these surface determinants. An example of multiple determinants can be found by close examination of the simple molecule bovine serum albumin (BSA).[2]

It has been estimated that there are approximately 60 distinct antigenic determinants that characterize the molecule of BSA and that the animal's response in making an anti-BSA antiserum is due to these 60 determinants. Therefore, what we call anti-BSA is really a collection of multiple antibodies directed to each of these determinants. Each of these antibodies is a product of a single or clone of plasma cells that can be found within the immunized animal. Hybridoma technology allows us to isolate each of these cells and create a small factory of antibody-producing cells that can be separated so that large quantities of the monoclonal antibody to a single antigenic determinant can be isolated. Each of these clones taken individually produce antibody directed to surface components, but this creates somewhat of a limitation because the distinction of major versus minor determinants cannot often be made when dealing with a monoclonal antibody as can be made when dealing with polyclonal antibodies to the antigen.

Another limiting feature of monoclonal antibodies is more evident in the use of cells such as lymphocytes, or virus-infected cells to produce a multiplicity of monoclonal antibodies directed to cell surface determinants. Often, our knowledge of the structure of various membrane components is limited and subtleties that were not previously evident using polyclonal antibody become more apparent utilizing monoclonal antibodies. Investigators have had to modify the conclusions as to what a membrane structure appears to be on the surface of the cell because of the use of monoclonal antibodies. Investigators using monoclonal antibodies are in the very early stages of probing membrane structures but the future is very promising.

With the availability of monoclonal antibodies becoming more accessible, laboratorians should beware of some of the significant technical limitations associated with these antibodies. Monoclonal antibodies are best used when the methodology focuses on the primary phase of an antibody-antigen reaction. Techniques such as immunofluorescence, radioimmunoassay, enzyme-immuno assay and immunoabsorbants are the best techniques to use with monoclonal antibodies. Those techniques commonly used by blood bankers such as agglutination and precipitation are methods which use the secondary phase of an antibody reaction to detect the presence of an antigen structure. Monoclonal antibodies are poor agglutinating and precipitating reagents.

Monoclonal Antibodies to Detect the Presence of Virus

One of the best examples of the power of the use of monoclonal antibodies is the study of viral antigens and cell-associated viral antigens. Because these virus-directed structures can clearly be dissected by isolating the products of an immune response from an animal, one should be able to detect subtle variations or generic drifts in viruses. One can also, in the proper experimental setting, use monoclonal antibodies to record the events or imprints a virus leaves upon a host cell when infection occurs. Monoclonal antibodies have been generated against influenza, para-influenza, rabies, herpes, measles, SV-40, reovirus, and RNA tumor viruses.

Using these monoclonal antibodies, it has been possible to identify substrates of many viruses that are a result of minor modification in virus protein and virus assembly. These monoclonal antibodies have helped to isolate many different variations of the same virus that were formerly undistinguishable with polyclonal antibodies. A good example is that traditional antibodies or polyclonal antibodies reveal no differences among rabies viruses isolated in different parts of the world.[3] These observations led to the belief that the antigenic characteristics of rabies were rather stable and that the virus used to produce various vaccines should provide adequate immunization anywhere in the world. Monoclonal antibodies, however, have divulged significant antigenic determinant differences among isolates from different parts of the world. This finding has raised the possibility that some vaccines will be failures due to the significant antigenic differences between various virus strains. With monoclonal antibodies, selection of more effective viral strains for the production of vaccines should be possible.

More recently, in our institutions, Smith and Murphy[4] have been evaluating various monoclonal antibodies directed against mouse cytomegalic virus (MCMV). Smith has been able to produce numerous monoclonal antibodies to a variety of antigenic determinants associated with the MCMV and the cell infected with MCMV. Many of these monoclonal antibodies seem to be recognizing various stages of cell infection in assembly of the virus. Within four hours of infection with the virus, there are already demonstrable changes that occur in the membrane of the cell. Some of these changes reflect development of Fc receptors but others are clearly new antigenic determinants that are derived because of the presence of virus. It was surprising to them to observe that these detectable changes in the membrane of the infected cell occurred as early as four hours after infection.

Previous to this, polyclonal antibody did not detect clearly these changes. It was only with the evolution or the development of monoclonal antibodies that these membrane structural changes were observed. They have also produced evidence using these monoclonal antibodies, that these membrane proteins are developed de novo as a result of virus infection of the cell. The function of these new membrane structures has yet to be elucidated. Other monoclonal antibodies these investigators have produced identify antigenic determinants exclusively associated with the nuclear membrane of an infected cell while others detect cytoplasmic antigenic determinants associated with the virus. It is conceivable with this wide variety of monoclonal antibodies that one may use these tools to isolate and characterize each of these structures and be able to create a temporal frame for the infection and replication of the virus in the cell. Monoclonal antibodies can also be raised against individual polypeptide chains of many different viruses that can be used to study the replication of virus and the relationship between the nonstructural and structural polypeptide chains.

Monoclonal Antibodies Against Parasites

Parasites can exist in many physical forms during their life cycles. Monoclonal antibodies should be able to be produced that recognize membrane structures of parasites during various stages in their life cycles. Monoclonal antibodies have been produced against surface glycoproteins of trypanosomes and have proved very useful in describing complex genetic and antigenic changes that occur in this organism. Significant progress has also been made in the study of malaria. It is known from studies using animal models immunized with sporozoites that the resultant antibody raised against surface antigen structures can neutralize the parasite. With monoclonal antibodies, it is possible to show that the sporozoite has six major components. One of these monoclonal antibodies has been shown to be specific for the parasite and for a particular stage in its life cycle. When the antibody is passively administered to infected animals, this antibody protects the animal from infection.

Monoclonal antibodies have also been prepared against different strains, and have been shown to interfere with the penetration of the parasite into the red blood cell. It is evident from these studies that monoclonal antibodies interfere with the development of the parasite and, thus, break the chain to protect effectively the animal against infection. By using monoclonal antibodies to probe the structure of various parasites, further understanding of their life cycle, as well as their most infectious stage, may be an important observation in the control of parasitic diseases in the world.

Monoclonal Antibodies Against Tumor Differentiation Antigens in Man

Generation of monoclonal antibodies have been successfully prepared against tumor antigens and a variety of cell surface glycoproteins on normal and malignant human lymphoid cells. Monoclonal antibodies have been prepared to a variety of polymorphic and nonpolymorphic antigens associated with thymic differentiation antigens, antigens specific for or associated with melanomas and leukemias, colorectal, breast, and lung cancer. The best example of application of monoclonal antibody technology in the probing of cell surface structures is found with the multiplicity of monoclonal antibodies prepared against human lymphocyte subpopulations.[6] Many of these monoclonal antibodies are currently available through commercial sources. These antibodies can recognize cells early in the development of the immune system in an individual. They characterize the prethymic, early thymic, and late thymic lymphocytes. They also characterize lymphoid populations as to their helper or suppressor cell function. These antibodies have been applied in a wide range of clinical settings in an attempt to define either the immune responses during a disease process, or to associate the disease process with an aberration in the immune system. A major question still facing investigators using these monoclonal antibodies to various T-lymphocyte subsets is to define that changes in the immune system in the various disease processes, and related phenotypic aberrations, truly also reflect a functional aberration in these cell populations. In some clinical situations, there is a direct relationship of the disease process with these aberrations. However, in numerous other clinical situations, the relationship to aberrations within lymphoid populations in the disease process must be further investigated.

The best application for monoclonal antibodies directed to lymphocyte populations has been found in the defining of immunodeficiency states and T-cell malignancies. In these situations, monoclonal antibodies have provided a clarification of the underlying disease processes. More recently, monoclonal antibodies directed to T-cells have been applied as therapeutic agents in the treatment of various T-cell malignancies. Although the results at this stage are very preliminary, there appears to be some promise in the utilization of these antibodies as therapeutic modalities. One foresees in the future the utilization of monoclonal antibodies linked to various cytotoxic drugs as a mechanism to focus the maximum amount of therapeutic agent in the tumor site itself. Monoclonal antibodies against solid tumor antigens may also be utilized as therapeutic agents but also may extend the diagnostic capabilities for identifying metastatic lesions by coupling biological tracers to the monoclonal antibodies.

Monoclonal Antibodies to the Major Histocompatibility Complex in Man

The central role of the major histocompatibility gene complex in a multiplicity of biological processes is now well established. It is apparent that better definition of gene products is needed. Monoclonal antibodies can provide a significantly new approach to the development of reagents capable of more specifically defining histocompatibility antigens in man. This will provide a better mechanism for the biochemical and immunochemical characterization of these antigens, which has been limited by the availability of high-titer reagents. The availability of monoclonal antibodies will permit the development of high titer and large quantities of specific antibody. To date, monoclonal antibodies have been produced to beta-2-microglobulin, to constant and polymorphic determinants of the HL-A, B, C, and DR loci, and to various components of the complement pathway which appear to be related to the major histocompatibility complex.[7] The development of these antibodies in sufficient quantity will also allow more appropriate standardization throughout the world related to the detection of antigens associated with the compatibility complex.

Summary

Hybridoma technology has produced a very powerful tool available to many scientific disciplines for the exploration of antigenic structures associated with the biologic membrane. These tools can be used to recognize subtle changes that occur within a virus-infected cell. They can be utilized in the development of more appropriate vaccines for the control of serious viral infections. The science of parasitology will be greatly enhanced by the utilization of monoclonal antibodies to investigate cell surface structures that occur on the parasite during its life cycle. This will allow further understanding of the genetics and receptor mechanisms associated with parasites involved in human disease. Monoclonal antibodies can also be utilized in the detection of cell differentiation antigens as well as describing cell function. The richest application in this area has occurred in defining both B- and T-lymphocyte subpopulations. In addition, tumor antigens previously detected utilizing polyclonal antibody now can be more specifically investigated with monoclonal antibodies. This potentially will allow a diagnostic and therapeutic approach in the future with specificity and sensitivity that hitherto had not been available. Finally, monoclonal antibody technology will play a very significant role in defining more specifically products of the major histocompatibility complex in man. This will provide the laboratorian and the clinical investigator with more powerful tools that potentially may allow us to manipulate the immune response in individuals and possibly modify various disease processes.

We presently are in the early stages of exploiting the potential of monoclonal antibodies and their application as probes to detect and characterize cell surface structures. This technology offers significant promise to a better understanding of cell surface structures that are important in the understanding and control of disease.

References

1. Kohler G, Milstein C. Continuous cultures of fused cells secreting antibody of predefined specificity. Nature 1975;256:495-7.
2. Habeeb AF, Atassi MZ. A fragment comprising the last third of bovine serum albumin which accounts for almost all the antigenic reactivity of native protein. J Biol Chem 1976;251:4616.
3. Witbor T. Monoclonal antibodies to rabies virus. Clin Immunol Newsletter 1980;1:1-5.
4. Murphy M, Smith R. (To be published.)
5. Immunological reviews: immunoparasitology. Vol 61, 1982.
6. Reinherz EL, Schlossman SF. The characterization and function of human immunoregulatory T-lymphocyte subsets. Immunology Today 1981;2:69-75.
7. Immunological reviews: hybrid myeloma monoclonal antibodies against MHC products. Vol. 47, 1979.

3

Nonisotopic Immunoassays in Blood Group Serology

Fred V. Plapp, MD, PhD, and Lyle T. Sinor, MT(ASCP)

Introduction

THE IMMUNOLOGICAL TECHNIQUE OF AGGLUTINATION was first discovered in 1888 by Stillmark when he observed that seed extracts of *Ricinus communis* strongly agglutinated erythrocytes.[1] In 1900, Ehrlich and Morgenroth reported that erythrocytes could also be agglutinated by alloantibodies.[2] Shortly thereafter, Landsteiner discovered the A, B and H blood group antigens using agglutination.[3] During the past 90 years, agglutination has remained the most widely used method in blood banking to detect the interaction of antibodies with cellular antigens. Other techniques, such as agglutination inhibition, antibody absorption and elution, complement fixation, immunofluorescence, and radioimmunoassay, have also been used on a much more limited basis.

More recently RBC, platelet, and neutrophil enzyme immunoassays (EIA) have been developed; however, their use has been largely restricted to detecting cell-associated IgG. This limited application of immunoassays in blood banking is in sharp contrast with the diverse application of these techniques in other areas of laboratory medicine such as: serology, virology, microbiology, endocrinology, toxicology, and clinical chemistry. In all of these areas, nonisotopic immunoassays, in particular, are extremely attractive because they offer the advantages of specificity, sensitivity, objective quantitation, and inexpensive automation. Because of these advantages it is estimated that greater than 50% of all clinical immunoassays will be nonisotopic by 1985. Since the future of nonisotopic immunoassays in clinical medicine appears so promising, the immunochemical principles

Fred V. Plapp, MD, PhD, Assistant Medical Director, Community Blood Center of Greater Kansas City, Kansas City, Missouri
Lyle T. Sinor, MT (ASCP), Graduate Student, University of Kansas Medical Center and Community Blood Center of Greater Kansas City, Kansas City, Missouri

underlying these techniques and their applicability to blood banking are presented.

The Evolution of Immunoassays

The widespread use of immunoassays for diagnostic purposes began with the development of fluorescent antibody-staining techniques in 1941 by Coons.[4] These immunofluorescent methods require the incubation of cells or tissue sections with antibodies directed toward a specific antigen. The antibody itself may be labeled with a fluorescent tag or, more frequently, it may be labeled indirectly by incubation with a labeled second antibody directed against the first antibody. These methods are very useful for the rapid identification of microorganisms as well as for the detection of antibodies present in infectious and autoimmune diseases. However, immunofluorescent methods suffer from being time-consuming, dependent upon subjective interpretation of results, and difficult to automate.

The introduction of radioimmunoassays (RIA) in 1959 by Yalow and Berson[5] further extended the clinical application of immunoassays. In this method, a purified antigen is labeled with a radioactive isotope and allowed to compete with unlabeled antigen present in the specimen for a limited number of antibody binding sites. The radioactivity of either the free or bound antigen is then determined after separation of these two antigen populations. These assays are extremely sensitive, specific, precise, and widely applicable to proteins, glycoproteins, drugs, and hormones. They are also amenable to automation for large scale processing. However, the use of isotopes has several serious disadvantages which include costly reagents with a short shelf-life, expensive counting equipment, the need to separate free from bound antigen prior to counting, and the health hazards associated with handling and disposal of radioactive wastes. These limitations have excluded RIA from many smaller laboratories.

Because of the inherent limitations with immunofluorescent assays and RIAs considerable effort has been expended to develop alternative labels for antibodies and antigens and to improve upon separation and detection techniques. This search has led to the development of numerous nonisotopic immunoassays. At present the most promising new nonisotopic labels are enzymes, which are covalently linked to antibodies, antigens, or Protein A such that the conjugates retain both immunologic and enzymatic activities. These enzyme conjugates can then act upon a variety of chromogenic, fluorigenic, or chemilumines-cent substrates. Other labels such as fluorophores, particles, and stable free radicals are also receiving increasing attention. Use of these labels eliminates the problems of reagent stability, safety, and high cost encountered with radioimmunoassay. Separation of bound from free enzyme conjugates has also been greatly simplified by immobilizing either the antigens or the antibodies on a solid phase, such as a plastic surface. This separation method is a key feature of all heterogeneous enzyme immunoassays. These assays are particularly suitable for the detection and measurement of high molecular weight (> 10,000) sub-stances, such as proteins.

Although immobilization on a solid phase greatly simplifies these assays, washing steps are still required which delay processing and increase the chance for error. For these reasons, homogeneous immunoassays have been developed which avoid separation steps. In these assays, antibody binding to antigen alters either enzymatic activity or fluorescence emission. This alteration allows the distinction of bound from free label without prior separation and allows increased speed, improved precision, and automation.

In the past, the use of homogeneous immunoassays has been limited to low molecular weight substances. However, new advances have extended their use to larger macromolecules. In all of these nonisotopic immunoassays, the final product can be measured with relatively in-expensive equipment. A comparison of homogeneous and hetero-geneous EIA with RIA and immunofluorescence is made in Table 1, and the advantages of EIAs are summarized in Table 2.

Types of Immunoassays

From the previous section, it can be seen that many different varieties of nonisotopic immunoassays can be designed. The final configuration depends on whether a heterogeneous or homogeneous assay is used, which component is labeled, and which label and substrate are chosen. The most commonly used heterogeneous and homogeneous assays are summarized in Tables 3 and 4.

As seen in Table 3, most of the heterogeneous nonisotopic immunoassays use enzymes as the label. Heterogeneous enzyme im-munoassays (EIA) have been given many synonymous names such as immunoassay, enzyme-linked immunoassay, enzyme-labeled immunoassay, immunoenzymatic assay and enzyme-linked immuno-

25

Table 1.—Comparison of Homogeneous and Heterogeneous EIA with RIA and Immunofluorescence

	Homogeneous EIA	Heterogeneous EIA	RIA	Immuno-fluorescence
Sensitivity	Low	High	Very high	High
Specificity	Dependent on antiserum quality			
Precision	Good	Good	Good	Low (semi-quantitative)
Complexity	Simple	Complex	Very complex	Complex
Assay Time	Minutes	Hours	Hours	Hours
License	None	None	Required	None
Equipment	Photometer	Photometer or naked eye	Isotope counter	Fluorescence microscope
Automation potential	Very high	High	Moderate	Low
Required expertise	Medium	Medium	High	High
Reagent stability	Good	Good	Poor	Variable

Table 2.—Advantages of Nonisotopic Immunoassay Methods

Wide applicability

Sensitive and specific

Inexpensive detection equipment

Inexpensive reagents with long shelf-lives

Simple and rapid protocols

Separation step may be eliminated

Potential for multiple, simultaneous assays
using different labels

Potential for automation

No radiation hazard

26

Table 3.—Heterogeneous Nonisotopic Immunoassays

Assay Type	Assay For	Immobilized Component	Labeled Component	Labels	Substrates	Detection
Competitive	Antigen	Antibody	Antigen	Enzymes;		
				Alkaline phosphatase	PNPP*	Colorimetry
					4MUP†	Fluorometry
				Peroxidase	DB‡	Colorimetry
					OPD§	Colorimetry
				Galactosidase	ONPG‖	Colorimetry
					4MUG¶	Fluorometry
Double antibody sandwich	Antigen	Antibody	Antibody	Enzymes	Any	Colorimetry
				Isoluminol	of	Luminometry
Modified double antibody sandwich	Antigen	Antibody	Anti-antibody	Enzymes	Above	Colorimetry Fluorometry
Indirect	Antibody	Antigen	Anti-antibody	Enzymes	Substrates	Colorimetry Fluorometry

* paranitrophenyl phosphate
† 4 methylumbelliferyl phosphate
‡ 3,3′ diaminobenzidine tetrahydrochloride

§ O-phenylenediamine
‖ O-nitrophenyl beta-galactopyranoside
¶ 4 methylumbelliferyl beta-D-galactoside

Table 4.—Homogeneous Nonisotopic Immunoassays

Assay Type	Label	Labeling Procedure	Detection
Enzyme multiplied immunoassay	Enzymes*	Simple to complicated	Colorimeter Luminometer Fluorometer
Fluorigenic substrate assays	Fluorescent substrate	Simple	Fluorometer
Fluorescent enhancement	Fluorophores†	Simple	Fluorometer
Fluorescent quenching	Fluorophores†	Simple	Fluorometer
Fluorescent polarization	Fluorophores†	Simple	Fluorometer
Fluorescent protection	Fluorophores†	Simple	Fluorometer
Energy transfer	Fluorescent donors and acceptors	Simple	Fluorometer
Spin immunoassay	Stable free radicals	Complicated	Electronic spin resonance
Particle counting immunoassay	Latex	Simple	Particle counter

* Dehydrogenases, lysozyme
† Fluorescein, rhodamine, fluorescamine, umbelliferone derivatives.

sorbent assay. The different types of enzyme immunoassays are described below,[6,7] and their chemical reactions are summarized in the Appendix.

Competitive EIA is a system for the detection and measurement of antigen. In this assay a specific antibody is attached to the solid phase which is then washed to remove unbound antibody. The specimen containing the antigen is then added along with enzyme-labeled antigen and allowed to incubate. During this incubation labeled antigen competes with unlabeled antigen for binding to the limited number of solid phase antibody molecules. Antibody-bound antigen is then separated from free antigen by washing. Enzyme substrate is added and a color reaction develops. The more antigen that is present in the specimen, the less labeled antigen that will be bound to the solid phase antibody and the smaller the color change produced. This procedure is analogous to classical RIA methods and is very sensitive. The primary disadvantages of this procedure are the need for abundant quantitites of pure antigen and the need to label each specific antigen.

An alternative EIA for detection of antigen is the double antibody sandwich method. In this assay, the solid phase is coated with excess specific antibody. This antibody is first reacted with the test sample containing the antigen and, after incubation and washing, the bound antigen is reacted with excess labeled specific antibody. After further washing, substrate is added and the color produced is measured. The amount of color produced is directly proportional to the amount of antigen. This technique is analogous to the immunoradiometric assay and has similar specificity and sensitivity for high molecular weight antigens. The antigen detected with this technique must be large enough to possess two antibody-binding sites. Each specific antibody used to detect a different antigen must be labeled.

A variation of the double antibody sandwich EIA employs a third antibody. Specific antibody produced in one animal is attached to the solid phase, washed, and incubated with the test sample containing the antigen. After washing, specific antibody to the antigen, which was produced in a different species than the first antibody, is incubated with the solid phase antibody-antigen complex. An enzyme labeled anti-Ig, reactive with only the second antibody, is then added. Finally, substrate is added and the color change is proportional to the amount of antigen in the sample. The advantage of this method is that it avoids labeling of each specific antibody.

The indirect ELISA measures antibody. In this method antigen is immobilized on the solid phase and incubated with test sera. Antibody present in the sample binds to the solid phase antigen which is present in excess. After washing an enzyme-labeled anti-Ig is added. This will bind to any antibody already attached to the antigen. The color change produced following substrate addition is proportional to the antibody concentration in the sera. This method is analogous to the classical indirect immunofluorescence assays described earlier and the radioallergosorbent (RAST) technique used for measuring reagins.

A modification of the indirect assay based on inhibition can also be used to measure antigens. The solid phase is coated with specific antigen and then incubated simultaneously with a mixture of the test sample and a reference antibody. If the sample does not contain antigen, the antibody binds to the solid phase antigen. If antigen is present in the sample, it combines with the antibody, which is then unable to bind to the solid phase antigen. The amount of antibody bound is measured by adding enzyme-labeled anti-Ig and substrate. The degree of inhibition of substrate degradation is proportional to the amount of the antigen in the sample.

Homogeneous enzyme immunoassays differ from heterogeneous assays because they do not require separation of free from bound label.[6-8] The enzyme multiplied immunoassay technique (EMIT) has been most widely used. Because these assays require only a mixing of reagents and subsequent measurement, they offer the possibilities of increased speed, simple instrumentation, and automation. In these immunoassays, a hapten is linked to an enzyme in such a manner that enzyme activity is either enhanced or inhibited following antibody binding to the hapten. To perform these assays, the test sample is mixed with the labeled hapten and with the specific antibody to the hapten. If hapten is present in the test sample it will compete with labeled hapten for the limiting number of antibody molecules. This competition results in less antibody being available to inhibit or activate the enzyme activity of the labeled hapten. The enzyme can hydrolyze chromogenic, fluorimetric, or chemiluminescent substrates. The latter two substrates theoretically provide increased sensitivity. However, in practice the sensitivity of most homogeneous assays using optical detection methods is limited by background interference such as absorbance or fluorescence of other substances in the sample. Generally, these assays are sensitive in the ng/ml range.

Until recently, homogeneous immunoassays were limited to the measurement of small haptens such as drugs and hormones. Antibody-induced modulation of the enzyme activity of the labeled hapten is due to conformational effects on the enzyme, caused by binding of the antibody to the enzyme-hapten. The binding of antibody to a small hapten permits a close interaction of the antibody with the enzyme. Antibody binding to a larger protein antigen-enzyme conjugate does not affect enzyme activity nearly as efficiently, since transmission of these conformational effects is attenuated by the large protein intervening between the antibody and the enzyme. This shortcoming has recently been overcome by coupling *E. coli* beta-galactosidase to proteins.[9] Antibody binding to protein beta-galactosidase conjugates causes steric exclusion of large substrate molecules from the active site and inhibits enzyme activity. This technique has been successfully applied to measurements of human IgG, IgM, and albumin in serum.[9]

The homogeneous substrate-labeled fluorescent immunoassay has also proven to be a useful technique for rapid quantitation of both low and high molecular weight substances.[10] This method has also been used to measure human immunoglobulins. This assay's sensitivity, reproducibility, and speed compare favorably with the enzyme-multipled immunoassay. This assay is based on the principle of competitive protein binding and requires three components: a fluorigenic label, an enzyme, and an antibody. The protein to be quantitated is covalently labeled with a fluorigenic enzyme substrate. The substrate, itself, is not fluorescent until it is hydrolyzed by the enzyme. When a specific antibody binds to the substrate-labeled protein, the substrate is no longer accessible to the enzyme and no fluorescence is produced. When protein is present in a test sample, it competes with the substrate-labeled protein for a limited number of antibody-binding sites and, therefore, less labeled protein is bound. Since more labeled protein is free to react with the enzyme, the fluorescence increases proportionally to the amount of protein in the test sample. The main disadvantage of this technique is that serum contains many components such as bilirubin, which also fluoresce and cause background interference.

The fluorescent properties of molecules are very susceptible to environmental influences. These influences have been taken advantage of in the development of a variety of new homogeneous fluorescent immunoassays which do not depend on enzymes to generate fluorescent products. The simplest of these assays involve the quenching or enhancement of a fluorescent label following antibody binding. Direct quenching fluorescent immunoassays rely on a decrease in the fluorescence of the labeled antigen following antibody binding while the free antigen exhibits full fluorescence.[11] This method is only suitable for haptens. However, an indirect quenching fluoroimmunoassay is suitable for proteins.[11] This technique utilizes two antibodies, one antibody is directed against the fluorescent label. In this technique, a pure population of the protein to be assayed is fluorescently labeled. The labeled protein is added to the test sample and then antibody specific for the protein is added. The protein in the sample competes with the labeled protein for a limited number of antibody-binding sites. If protein is present in the sample, it binds to the antibody and a corresponding amount of labeled protein remains unbound. Anti-fluorescent label antibodies are then added and bind to the free labeled protein. This binding quenches the fluorescent label. The anti-fluorescent label antibody is sterically hindered from binding to the labeled protein which is already bound to the antiprotein antibody. Therefore, if little protein is present in the sample, most of the labeled protein will be bound by antiprotein antibody and will not react with antifluorescent label antibody so that a high fluorescence level will remain. These assays are also known as fluorescent protection immunoassays since binding to the first antibody protects the fluorescent label. In the future, this approach may also be feasible using enzymes as labels, since antibodies can easily be made against enzymes.

Fluorescent polarization immunoassay (FPIA) was first developed by Dandliker et al[12] in 1973. However, this technique has not been widely accepted in clinical laboratories due to the expensive and complicated instrumentation required for measurement. This problem may be solved with the recent development of simple and inexpensive instruments,[13] and the demonstration that this technique can be used for therapeutic drug monitoring. FPIA uses a fluorescently labeled antigen and a specific antibody in a competitive-binding homogeneous immunoassay. The labeled antigen competes for antibody-binding sites with unlabeled antigen present in the sample. Detection of free and bound antigen depends on the Brownian movement of the fluorescent particles. When labeled antigens are free in solution, they rotate rapidly so that different molecules are more likely to have a random orientation at any point in time. When these randomly oriented molecules are excited by linear polarized light they emit depolarized light. However, when the fluorescent antigen binds to antibody, the fluorescent label is constrained and rotates much more slowly so that the molecules remain polarized between the times that light is absorbed and emitted. When linearly polarized light excites the bound fluorescent label, the emitted light is still polarized. The greater the concentration of an antigen in a specimen, the smaller the amount of fluorescent label that is bound by antibody and the less polarization obtained. The applicability of this technique for measurement of macromolecules remains to be seen.

Another homogeneous immunoassay that is applicable to the assay of a wide range of haptens and protein antigens is fluorescence excitation transfer immunoassay.[14] This assay measures antibody-antigen binding by detecting the dipole-dipole coupled electronic energy transfer that occurs when an antigen labeled with a fluorescent energy donor (fluorescer) comes into close proximity with an antibody labeled with a fluorescent energy acceptor (quencher). Antigen in solution is fluorescent but this fluorescence is quenched following antibody binding. The immunoassay is performed by mixing a fluorescer-antigen and a quencher-antibody with the test specimen. Competitive binding by the unlabeled antigen in the specimen for antibody-binding sites will inhibit the binding of fluorescer-antigen and lead to an increase in fluorescent intensity.

An alternative method using only labeled antibody can be performed if a large antigen is being assayed.[14] This method entails labeling one portion of a highly purified antibody with a fluorescent donor and a second portion of the same antibody with a nonfluorescent acceptor. Both of these labeled antibodies are added to sample being tested. If antigen is present both antibodies will bind to the large antigen in close enough proximity for dipole-coupled energy transfer to occur. This will result in fluorescence quenching and a decrease in fluorescence intensity. This method requires highly purified fluorescer-labeled antibody in order to avoid high background fluorescence which would mask fluorescence quenching. The other potential problem with this assay is that if a sample has excess antigen compared to antibody, the fluorescer and quencher antibodies are more likely to bind to separate antigen molecules rather than the same molecule, preventing fluorescent quenching. In practice, an assay requires 50% quenching of fluorescer-labeled antigen or antibody to be useful.

Latex particle agglutination has been a widely used serological technique since its introduction for detection of rheumatoid factor in 1956.[15] This technique is simple and has been widely applied for the detection of antigens, antibodies, and immune complexes. The limitations of this method are the difficulty in determining an objective end point and nonspecific interference of agglutination by serum components unrelated to the antigen-antibody system being measured. Recently, a particle-counting immunoassay has been developed which avoids these pitfalls and provides increased sensitivity and complete automation.[16] This immunoassay is based on the principle that the number of free particles decreases following agglutination and this decrease can be readily detected with a particle counter. For instance, antigen in a test sample can be quantitated by mixing the sample with latex beads coated with a specific antibody. If antigen is present, it will agglutinate the antibody-coated beads, resulting in a decreased number of free particles. This method has a sensitivity of 0.1-1.0 ng/ml for most proteins and has been widely applied to the measurement of hormones, immunoglobulins, viruses, bacteria, parasites, and other serum proteins.

Spin immunoassays are based on the observation that the electron spin resonance signal of a hapten labeled with a stable free radical changes following binding of a specific antibody.[17] This assay is limited in its applicability because of its complexity, expense, and lack of sensitivity.

Practical Aspects

Solid Phase

All of the heterogeneous and some of the homogeneous immunoassays employ either antigen or antibody immobilized on a solid phase. Particulate beads synthesized from cellulose, agarose, dextran, polyacrylamide, nylon, or glass are suitable. However, they require covalent coupling of proteins with carbodiimides and repeated centrifugation in the washing steps of the assay. These steps are inconvenient and time-consuming. The use of tubes or microtiter plates for the solid phase obviates the need for centrifugation and simplifies handling of large numbers of tests because washing is accomplished by merely filling and decanting. Microtiter plates are most commonly used because they minimize reagent volumes and are more amenable to total automation. Plates, tubes, and beads molded from polystyrene, polypropylene, and polyvinyl plastics have all been used successfully. They have the added advantage that protein can be coupled simply by passive adsorption. Passive adsorption is believed to occur by hydrophobic bonds.[18] Polystyrene has been used most frequently since it reproducibly adsorbs adequate quantities of antibody or antigen. The optimal conditions for passive adsorption of protein to plastic should be investigated for each individual application.[18,19] However, in general, most proteins and lipoproteins react best at a concentration of 1-10 μg/ml when suspended in buffer at pH 9.6. Adsorption occurs rapidly, reaching completion within two to four hours at room temperature or overnight at 4 C. When binding antibody to plastic, the Ig fraction, rather than crude antiserum, should be used to increase the amount of specific antibody bound per surface area. Similarly, relatively pure antigen fractions should be used for binding. For all protein studies to date, the saturation limit of protein binding has been about 1 μg of protein per cm^2 of plastic surface.[18,19] Therefore, addition of protein concentrations greater than 10 μg/ml for adsorption is wasteful.

In an attempt to covalently bind proteins to plastic surfaces, some authors have pretreated the plastic with glutaraldehyde immediately prior to the addition of the protein.[19] The protein is then added in neutral phosphate-buffered saline at a concentration of 10-100 μg/ml and incubated overnight. The plates are then washed with buffer-containing gelatin to block any unreacted glutaraldehyde. This method increases the amount of protein bound twofold, but may decrease the antigen-binding capacity of some antibodies.

Recently, methods have also been described to bind bacterial and eucaryotic cells directly to plastic. Small cells[20] and membrane vesicles[21] will passively adsorb directly to plastic, whereas larger cells require an anchor for firm attachment. Poly-L-lysine, a large polycationic molecule, has been most successfully used for this purpose.[20,22] Poly-L-lysine adheres tightly to plastic, leaving free cationic sites which can attach to negatively charged cell surfaces. The cells are then fixed in place by treatment with glutaraldehyde. Fixation with dilute glutaraldehyde solutions does not alter the antigenicity of cells.[20] These plates can be stored for months without loss of antigen activity.

Enzyme Conjugates

The heterogeneous and homogeneous enzyme linked immunoassays all require either an antibody-enzyme or antigen-enzyme conjugate. Criteria which should be considered in choosing an enzyme for conjugation are listed in Table 5.

Table 5.—Criteria for Choosing an Enzyme

1. Inexpensive and readily available in purified form.
2. High specific activity.
3. Stable during storage and assay.
4. Soluble in aqueous buffers.
5. Assay method that is simple, inexpensive, rapid, sensitive, and not affected by factors in biological fluids.
6. Contains reactive residues for chemical cross-linking.
7. Retains enzyme activity after conjugation.
8. Absent from biological fluids and cells being tested.
9. Enzyme, substrates, and cofactors are safe.
10. For homogeneous EIA: enzyme activity is enhanced or diminished by antibody binding.

Although many different enzymes have been tried, very few enzymes meet all of these requirements. Most heterogeneous EIAs use alkaline phosphatase, horseradish peroxidase, or beta-D-galactosidase since they meet most of these criteria.[6,7] Homogeneous EIAs for haptens most commonly use malate dehydrogenase, glucose-6-phosphate dehydrogenase, and lysozyme since these activities are modulated by antibody binding.[6,7] Homogeneous EIAs for proteins use beta-D-galactosidase.[9]

Although many methods exist to prepare protein-protein conjugates, only a few of these methods have been successfully used to produce enzyme-antibody conjugates.[23,24] The most successful methods are listed in Table 6.

Table 6.—Enzyme-Antibody Conjugation Methods

---

1. One-step glutaraldehyde.
2. Two-step glutaraldehyde.
3. Periodate oxidation.
4. N, N'-O-Phenylenedimaleimide
5. m-Maleimidobenzoyl-N-hydroxysuccinimide.

Glutaraldehyde is a dialdehyde that reacts with free amino groups in proteins to form a Schiff's base. The one-step glutaraldehyde method simply involves incubating a mixture of enzyme and antibody in the presence of glutaraldehyde until conjugation occurs, and then dialyzing to remove unreacted glutaraldehyde. This method is used frequently to couple alkaline phosphatase and horseradish peroxidase to antibodies. This method has several limitations. Antibody-antibody and enzyme-enzyme conjugates form in addition to the desired enzyme-antibody conjugate. The degree of conjugation is difficult to control so that large antibody-enzyme polymers occur. The efficiency of enzyme coupling is low so that only about 5% of the initial enzyme may be coupled. Also, antibody activity may be diminished by glutaraldehyde. In spite of these difficulties, the simplicity of this method has led to its widespread use for preparation of alkaline phosphatase-antibody conjugates.

The problems associated with the one-step method have led to the development of a two-step glutaraldehyde method for the coupling of horseradish peroxidase to antibody. This method yields conjugates which have an equal ratio of enzyme and antibody. This method takes advantage of the fact that each molecule of horseradish peroxidase binds only one aldehyde group preventing formation of enzyme-enzyme conjugates. Therefore, in this method peroxidase is preincubated with glutaraldehyde and the activated enzyme is separated from free glutaraldehyde before adding antibody. Antibody molecules couple only with activated peroxidase yielding conjugates consisting of one molecule of antibody and one molecule of antigen. The efficiency of enzyme coupling is as low as in the one-step method, but the lower molecular weight conjugates often result in increased sensitivity.

The periodate coupling method is also limited to horseradish peroxidase, but it gives better enzyme-coupling efficiency than the previous two methods. Horseradish peroxidase is a glycoprotein and the carbohydrate moiety can be oxidized by periodate to form aldehydes. These aldehyde groups react with free amino groups in the antibody molecules. This method results in 68% incorporation of the initial enzyme activity and 99% of the antibody into conjugates. These conjugates give much better dose-response curves in EIAs than do the previous methods, but the coupling procedure is more complicated.

N, N'-O-Phenylenedimaleimide is a homobifunctional reagent that couples proteins via their sulfhydryl groups. Sulfhydryl groups are first produced in Igs by mild reduction of disulfide bonds. These sulfhydryl groups then react with maleimide and the excess maleimide is removed by gel filtration. Activated Igs are then coupled to beta-D-galactosidase. This method efficiently couples enzyme to antibody with little loss of enzyme or antibody activity. Low molecular weight conjugates are formed. The coupling method is more complicated, but should be applicable to any enzymes containing free sulfhydryl groups. To date, only beta-D-galactosidase has been successfully used with this method.

Maleimidobenzoyl-N-hydroxysuccinimide ester (MBS) is a heterobifunctional reagent which has also been used to couple beta-D-galactosidase to antibodies. This procedure is simple and just as efficient as the phenylenedimaleimide method. The hydroxysuccinimide ester reacts with amino groups on nonreduced antibodies while the maleimide reacts with free sulfhydryl groups present in beta-D-galactosidase. Low molecular weight conjugates are formed. This method will probably receive increasing attention in the future since beta-D-galactosidase conjugates are very sensitive; this enzyme is not present in biological fluids, and both chromogenic and fluorigenic substrates are available. Also, this enzyme can be used in homogeneous EIAs for proteins.

All of these conjugates are stable for up to one year at 4 C. Many of them are also available commercially and have high specific activities. Often they can be diluted more than 1/1000, defraying the cost.

Substrates

The most commonly used substrates for these enzymes have already been listed in Table 3. For alkaline phosphatase, p-nitrophenyl phosphate is very sensitive and readily available commercially in preweighed tablets.[25] The colored product is measured at 405 nm. This substrate is sensitive enough for most immunoassays, but 4 methylumbelliferyl phosphate, which yields a fluorescent product, can be used to increase sensitivity.

Numerous substrates for horseradish peroxidase are available.[25] Many of these are not very soluble in water and are potential health hazards. Benzidine has been reported to be carcinogenic. O-Phenylenediamine appears to be the best substrate because it is readily soluble and has a high extinction coefficient at 494 nm. 2,3'-Azinodi(3-ethylbenzthiazoline-6-sulfonate) is less sensitive but more stable in light, and can also be used.[24,25]

The choice of substrates for beta-D-galactosidase is more limited since only one chromogenic (O-nitrophenyl beta-D-galactopyranoside)[25] and one fluorigenic (4-methylumbelliferyl beta-D-galactoside)[27] substrate are commercially available. Both of these substrates are very sensitive. The chromogenic product is measured at 420 nm while the fluorigenic product is excited at 360 nm and measured at 450 nm.

Fluorescent Labels

In general, most of the homogeneous fluorescent immunoassays have used fluorescein isothiocyanate (FITC) to label antigens. This label has been used successfully in the indirect quenching fluoroimmunoassays and fluorescent protection immunoassays.[11] Fluorescein conjugation is accomplished easily by mixing the antigen with an equal volume of FITC solution overnight and then removing residual unreacted FITC.[11] The emission wavelength of fluorescein is 575 nm. At this wavelength, there is little background fluorescence from serum factors, which emit between 400-490 nm.

Some of the other homogeneous fluorescent immunoassays require the synthesis of special derivatives of fluorescein. For instance, the fluorescers used in fluorescent excitation transfer immunoassays are N-hydroxysuccinimide esters of fluorescein, while the quenchers are 4', 5'-dimethoxyfluoresceins.[14] Likewise, fluorescent polarization techniques often use fluorescein derivatives. The homogeneous substrate-labeled fluorescent immunoassays utilize beta-D-galactosidase as the enzyme and a derivative of galactosylumbelliferone as the fluorigenic substrate.[10] The exact derivative used and the conjugation to antigen will have to be especially adapted for each new application. Umbelliferone has an emission wavelength of 450 nm, which leads to greater background fluorescence than encountered with fluorescein.

Detection and Automation

Most of these assays use an inexpensive spectrophotometer or fluorometer for quantitation of results. Spectrophotometers are also available which automatically read microtiter plates.[25,28] These spectrophotometers can be interfaced to printers, calculators, and minicomputers for data reduction. Assays performed in microtiter plates can be further automated by using automatic dispensers and washers. All of these instruments are commercially available. Results can be expressed in many ways, such as, positive or negative, an absorbance value, concentration, titer, or ratio of unknown to control.

Application to Blood Group Serology

As mentioned earlier the application of nonisotopic immunoassays to blood group serology has been limited to the detection of cell-bound immunoglobulins. Several assays have been described for detecting RBC-[29-32] and platelet-[33] associated immunoglobulin. By adapting the techniques described in the previous section, it should be possible to design simpler and faster assays for routine use in blood banking. This section will discuss some of these potential applications.

Recently, a competitive EIA has been used to detect platelet associated IgG in patients with idiopathic thrombocytopenic purpura.[34] In this assay enzyme-labeled anti-IgG binds to either platelet-associated IgG or to solid phase IgG. This assay is faster than other EIAs since it employs a solid phase and is more sensitive since it directly measures antibody on platelets. This method should also be applicable to quantitate RBC, neutrophil, and lymphocyte antibodies.

The modified double antibody sandwich EIA is useful for antigen typing of lymphocytes, RBCs, and platelets. Specific antibody is attached to microtiter plates and cells containing the appropriate antigen are then bound. The cells are detected by sequentially adding a second antibody and enzyme-labeled anti-IgG. This method allows large-scale screening of cellular antigens.

The indirect EIA is commonly used to screen monoclonal antibodies and to quantitate antiplatelet and antineutrophil antibodies in patients' sera.[35] In this latter application, glutaraldehyde-fixed platelets and neutrophils are passively adsorbed to microtiter plates. These solid phase cells are then incubated with the patient's serum, washed, and incubated with enzyme-labeled anti-IgG. A colored product indicates the presence of antibody. This assay is easily adaptable to RBC antibody screening. Intact RBCs or RBC membranes containing various antigen combinations are attached to microtiter plates, incubated with patient's serum, and then incubated with enzyme-labeled anti-IgG or anti-IgM. Our laboratory has demonstrated that RBC membranes attached to plastic retain their specificity for A, B, M, N, and Rh antibodies (unpublished observations). Antibody panels could also be devised using this method. Glutaraldehyde fixation of the solid phase cells would allow prolonged storage of these plates. Solid phase panels for antibody identification could be made more specific and easier to interpret by attaching purified membrane antigens to plastic. Fromageot[36] has demonstrated that the glycophorin A adsorbed to polystyrene retains its M, N specificity.

The rapidity and simplicity of homogeneous immunoassays make them particularly attractive for many routine blood banking procedures. The enzyme multiplied immunoassay technique (EMIT) might be useful for ABO and Rh typing if AB-positive RBCs were labeled with beta-galactosidase and the binding of anti-A, -B, or -D inhibited enzyme activity. Donor or recipient RBCs would be mixed with enzyme-labeled RBCs and typing serum would then be added. If the donor or recipient's RBCs contained the corresponding antigen, they would bind the antibody and enzyme activity would not be affected. If the RBCs lacked the antigen, antibody would bind to the enzyme-labeled RBC and inhibit enzyme activity. This assay could also be used for antibody screening by enzyme-labeling the RBC screening cells. If antibody was present in a patient's or donor's serum it would bind to the RBCs and inhibit enzyme activity.

In a similar fashion, the homogeneous substrate labeled fluorescent immunoassay could be used in routine blood banking. In this assay, RBCs would be labeled with a fluorescent substrate instead of an enzyme. The substrate itself is not fluorescent until it is cleaved by an enzyme. These labeled RBCs would be mixed with the donor or recipient RBCs, anti-A, -B, or -D, and an enzyme. If the unknown RBCs lack the antigen being tested for, all antibody will bind to the labeled RBCs and prevent the enzyme from cleaving the fluorescent substrate. Therefore, no fluorescence would be produced. On the other hand, if the RBCs possess the antigen they will bind antibody so that the substrate labeled RBCs remain accessible to the enzyme and fluorescence is observed. This assay could also be used for antibody screening if screening cells were labeled with fluorescent substrate.

The fluorescent excitation transfer immunoassay might be particularly well-suited for ABO and Rh typing. For instance, in order to type RBCs for A antigen one portion of an anti-A antibody would be labeled with a fluorescer while another portion would be labeled with a fluorescent quencher. The fluorescer itself is brightly fluorescent. However, if type A RBCs are added, the fluorescer-anti A and the quencher-anti A would bind to the RBC in close enough proximity to quench the fluorescence.

Particle-counting immunoassays are readily adaptable to identification of cell surface antigens.[37] These assays are very similar to rosette tests, which have been used for years to identify subpopulations of cells, except that they substitute latex beads for sheep RBCs. Latex beads could be coated with a specific antibody and allowed to react with unknown RBCs. If these RBCs possess the corresponding antigen they will bind to the latex beads, forming a larger agglutinated particle. The extent of agglutination can then be determined by either measuring the decrease in free RBCs or the increase in large agglutinated particles. Relatively inexpensive instruments are commercially available which can make both types of measurements. ABO and Rh typing, as well as antibody screening could be easily performed with this assay technique. A more sophisticated alternative to particle counting is the use of antibody-coated fluorescent latex beads and either a fluorometer or a fluorescent activated cell sorter.[38] Routine blood banking procedures probably do not require the increased sensitivity offered by using fluorescent immunospheres. Also, fluorescent detectors are considerably more complicated and expensive than particle counters.

Another aspect of ELISA technology that is useful in blood group serology is the use of solid phase antibodies to separate cell subpopulations. These techniques have been successfully used to separate T- and B-lymphocytes.[39] In this technique, antibody is passively adsorbed to plastic petri dishes and a mixture of cells is allowed to settle onto the bottom of the dish. Cells lacking the appropriate antigen are readily removed by washing, while cells containing the antigen remain bound to the dish. The adherent cells can then be harvested by vigorous agitation. The authors' laboratory has successfully used this simple technique to separate Tn-activated RBCs from normal RBCs (published observations). Other applications might include separation of fetal from maternal RBCs and separation of antibody-coated RBCs from normal RBCs.

Conclusion

As can be seen from the preceding discussion, a multitude of possibilities exist for the application of nonisotopic immunoassays to blood group serology. Although these immunoassays may appear too complicated and cumbersome at first, their methodologies will become

41

simpler and faster with increasing use. The application of nonistopic immunoassays to blood group serology will only be limited by our imagination and perseverence. We truly expect that one of these immunoassays will serve as a prototype for automated blood banking procedures in the future.

Appendix: Reaction Equations

Chemical Reactions of EIAs

Competitive EIA

$$\begin{matrix} \vdash Ab \\ \vdash Ab \end{matrix} + Ag - E + Ag \longrightarrow \begin{matrix} \vdash Ab \cdot Ag\text{-}E \\ \vdash Ab \cdot Ag \end{matrix}$$

Double Ab sandwich

$$\vdash Ab + Ag \longrightarrow \vdash Ab \cdot Ag + Ab\text{-}E \longrightarrow \vdash Ab \cdot Ag \cdot Ab\text{-}E$$

Modified double Ab sandwich

$$\vdash Ab^1 + Ag \longrightarrow \vdash Ab^1 \cdot Ag + Ab^2 \longrightarrow \vdash Ab^1 \cdot Ag \cdot Ab^2 + Ab^2\text{-}E \longrightarrow \vdash Ab^1 \cdot Ag \cdot Ab^2 \cdot anti\ Ab^2\text{-}E$$

Indirect EIA

$$\vdash Ag + Ab \longrightarrow \vdash Ag \cdot Ab + anti\ Ab\text{-}E \longrightarrow \vdash Ag \cdot Ab \cdot anti\ Ab\text{-}E$$

Modified indirect EIA

$$\vdash Ag + Ag + Ab \longrightarrow \vdash Ag \cdot Ab + anti\ Ab\text{-}E \longrightarrow \vdash Ag \cdot Ab \cdot Ag \cdot Ab \cdot anti\ Ab\text{-}E$$

EMIT

$$Ag\text{-}E + Ab \longrightarrow E\text{-}Ag \cdot Ab\ (altered\ enzyme\ activity)$$

$$Ag\text{-}E + Ag + Ab \longrightarrow E\text{-}Ag + Ag \cdot Ab\ (enzyme\ activity\ unaffected)$$

Homogeneous Substrate Labeled Fluorescent Immunoassay

$$\text{Ag-F}_{\text{substrate}} + \text{Ab} \xrightarrow{\text{enzyme}} \text{Ag-F}_{\text{substrate}} \cdot \text{Ab (no fluorescence)}$$

$$\text{Ag-F}_{\text{substrate}} + \text{Ag} + \text{Ab} \xrightarrow{\text{enzyme}} \text{Ag-F}_{\text{product}} + \text{Ag} \cdot \text{Ab (fluorescence)}$$

Indirect Fluorescent Quenching Immunoassay

Protein-Fl + anti-protein $\longrightarrow$ Fl-protein · anti-protein +
anti-Fl $\longrightarrow$ Fl-protein − anti-protein + anti-Fl (fluorescent)

Protein-Fl + protein + anti-protein $\longrightarrow$ protein · anti-protein +
protein-Fl + anti-Fl $\longrightarrow$ Fl-protein · anti-Fl (no fluorescence) +
protein · anti-protein

Fluorescence Excitation Transfer Immunoassay

Method 1

Ab-Q $\longrightarrow$ Ab-Q + Ag-F $\longrightarrow$ Q-Ab · Ag-F (not fluorescent)

Ab-Q + Ag $\longrightarrow$ Q-Ab · Ag + Ag + Ag-F $\longrightarrow$ Q-Ab · Ag +
Ag-F (fluorescent)

Method 2

$$\text{Ag} + \text{Ab-Q} + \text{Ab-F} \longrightarrow \text{Ag} \begin{array}{c} .\text{Ab-Q} \\ .\text{Ab-F} \end{array} \text{(not fluorescent)}$$

References

1. Stillmark H. Uber Ricin, ein giftiges Ferment aus den Samen von *Ricinus communis* L. and einigen anderen Euphorbiaceen, thesis. Dorpat, 1888.
2. Ehrlich P, Morgenroth J. Uber Haemolysine. Dritte Mitteilung. Berl Klin Wschr 1900;37:453-7.
3. Landsteiner K. Zur Kenntnis der antifermentattiven, lytischen und agglutinierenden Wirkungen des Blutserums und der Lymphe. Zbl Bakt 1900;27:357-62.
4. Coons AH, Creech HJ, Jones RN. Immunological properties of an antibody containing a fluorescent group. Proc Soc Exp Biol Med 1941;47:200-8.

5. Berson SA, Yalow RS. Quantitative aspects of the reaction between insulin and insulin-binding antibody. J Clin Invest 1959;38: 1996-2016.
6. Voller A, Bartlett A, Bidwell DE. Enzyme immunoassays with special reference to ELISA techniques. J. Clin Pathol 1978;31: 507-20.
7. Wisdom GB. Enzyme-immunoassay. Clin Chem 1976;22:1243-55.
8. Rubenstein K, Schneider R, Ullman E. Homogeneous enzyme immunoassay a new immunochemical technique. Biochem Biophy Res Commun 1972;47:846-51.
9. Gibbons I, Skold C, Rowley GL, Ullman EF. Homogeneous enzyme immunoassay for proteins employing B-galactosidase. Anal Biochem 1980;102:167-70.
10. Burd JF. The homogeneous substrate-labeled fluorescent immunoassay. Methods Enzymol 1981;74:79-87.
11. Nargessi RD, Landon J. Indirect quenching fluoroimmunoassay. Methods Enzymol 1981;74:60-85.
12. Dandliker WB, Kelly RJ, Dandliker J. Fluorescent polarization immunoassay. Theory and experimental method. Immunochemistry 1973;10:219-27.
13. Popelka R, Miller DM, Holen JT, Kelso DM. Fluorescence polarization immunoassay II. Clin Chem 1981;27:1198-201.
14. Ullman EF, Khanna PL. Fluorescence excitation transfer immunoassay. Methods Enzymol 1981;74:28-59.
15. Singer JM, Plotz CM. The latex fixation test: application to the serological diagnosis of rheumatoid arthritis. Am J Med 1956; 21:888-92.
16. Masson PL, Cambiaso CL, Collet-Cassart D, Magnusson CGM, Richards CB, Sindic CJM. Particle counting immunoassay. Methods Enzymol 1981;74:106-39.
17. Yang GC, Copeland ES. Spin immunoassay. Methods Enzymol 1981;74:140-51.
18. Herrman JE, Collins MF. Quantitation of immunoglobulin adsorption to plastics. J Immunol Methods 1976;10:363-6.
19. Parsons GE. Antibody-coated plastic tubes in radioimmunoassay. Methods Enzymol 1981;73:224-44.
20. Heusser CH, Stocker JW, Gisler RH. Methods for binding cells to plastic: application to solid phase immunoassays for cell surface antigens. Methods Enzymol 1981;73:406-18.
21. Sogin DC, Hinkle PC. Immunological identification of the human erythrocyte glucose transporter. Proc Natl Acad Sci USA 1980; 77:5725-9.

22. Polin RA, Kennett R. Use of monoclonal antibodies in an enzyme-linked inhibition assay for rapid detection of streptococcal antigen. J Ped 1980;97:540-4.
23. Avrameas S, Ternynck T, Guesdon JL. Coupling of enzymes to antibodies and antigens. Scand Immunol 1978;8(suppl 7):7-23.
24. O'Sullivan MJ, Marks V. Methods for the preparation of enzyme-antibody conjugates for use in enzyme immunoassay. Methods Enzymol 1981;73:147-65.
25. Voller A, Bidwell DE, Bartlett A. The enzyme linked immunosorbent assay (ELISA). Alexandria: Dynatech Laboratories, 1979.
26. Borzini P et al. An immunoenzymatic assay for the detection and quantitation of platelet antibodies: the platelet B-galactosidase test. J Immunol Methods 1981;44:323-32.
27. Ishikawa E, Kato K. Ultrasensitive enzyme immunoassay. Scan J Immunol 1978;8(suppl 7):43-55.
28. Saunders GC, Campbell S, Sanders WM, Martinez A. Automation and semiautomation of enzyme immunoassay instrumentation. In: Nakamura RM, Tucker ES, eds. Immunoassays in the clinical laboratory. New York: Alan R. Liss, 1979:119-38.
29. Bruner KW, Kissling CW. An enzyme linked immunosorbent assay (ELISA) for detecting IgG sensitized erythrocytes. Transfusion 1979;19:773-7.
30. Leikola J, Perkins HA. Enzyme-linked antiglobulin test: an accurate and simple method to quantify red cell antibodies. Transfusion 1980;20:138-44.
31. Osborne WRA, Giblett ER. Enzyme-linked immunosorbent assay for the anti-human globulin test. Acta Hematol 1980;63:124-7.
32. Gilman GE, Kennedy MS, Lott JA, Powers JD, Waheed A, Senhauser DA. Further improvement of the enzyme-linked antiglobulin test (ELAT) for erythrocyte antibodies. Am J Clin Pathol 1982;77:206-10.
33. Karpatkin S. Autoimmune thrombocytopenic purpura. Blood 1980;56:329-43.
34. Tsubakio T, Yoshiyuki K, Yonezawa T, Kitani T. Quantification of platelet-associated IgG with competitive solid-phase enzyme immunoassay. Acta Hemtol 1981;66:251-6.
35. Doughty R, Virge J, Magee J. An enzyme linked immunosorbent assay for leukocyte and platelet antibodies. J Immunol Methods 1981;47:161-9.
36. Fromageot HPM. Adsorption of human erythrocyte surface glycoprotein onto polystyrene latex spheres. J Lab Clin Med 1977;90:324-9.

37. Gabrilovac J, Pachmann K, Rodt H, Jage G, Thierfelder S. Particle-labeled antibodies. I. Anti-T cell antibodies attached to plastic beads by Poly-L-Lysine. J Immunol Methods 1979;30:161-70.
38. Higgins TJ, O'Neill HC, Parish CR. A sensitive and quantitative fluorescence assay for cell surface antigens. J Immunol Methods 1981;47:275-87.
39. Wysocki W, Sato VL. Panning for lymphocytes: a method for cell selection. Proc Natl Acad Sci USA 1978;75:2844-8.

4

Antibody Uptake: The First Stage of the Hemagglutination Reaction

B. P. L. Moore, DSc, MD

Introduction

WE SEEM, "TO HAVE MADE APPRECIABLE progress towards an orderly arrangement of evidence and a generalization of theory, which has resulted in a clearer conception of the processes involved." (Topley and Wilson's *Principles of Bacteriology and Immunity*, 1946[1]).

The first description of the agglutination reaction dealt with the flocculation of bacteria and appeared in 1896,[1] five years before the first human blood groups were discovered. For the first three decades of this century, most of our knowledge of this phenomenon came from the work of bacteriologists. Latterly, with the development of Immunology and the emergence of Immunochemistry, a "clearer concept of the processes involved" has slowly unfolded. And, although supported in part by experimental evidence, a concept it remains.

The variant with which we are here concerned, hemagglutination, is essentially an artificial phenomenon that takes place only in the laboratory. There are two stages which occur consecutively and concurrently, but reach maxima within different time-frames:

• First Stage or Stage of Combination: This is the stage of recognition of antigen by antibody. It occurs when an antibody molecule attaches to a specific site on the red cell membrane. The results are not directly observable.

• Second Stage or Stage of Coalescence: This is the stage of cell:cell interactions. It is the result of random collisions between antibody-coated cells which lead to crosslinkages between them by means of "bridges" of antibody molecules. The results are observable.

B. P. L. Moore, DSc, MD, Director, National Reference Laboratory, Canadian Red Cross Blood Transfusion Service, Toronto, Canada

Definitions

Blood Group Antigens

These may be protein, carbohydrate, or lipid, ie, they may be glycoprotein, lipoprotein, or glycolipid. With the exception of the extrinsic antigens Lewis, Chido, and Rodgers, which are introduced onto the cell membrane by adsorption from the plasma, they are intrinsic, integral components of the red cell membrane.

Antigenic Determinants

These are the minimal chemical subunits of antigen against which an antibody can be formed; as will be seen later, they also act as receptors for antibody-combining sites. An antigenic determinant may be as small as a single sugar residue or as large as six sugar or nine amino-acid residues.[2] In a protein, a determinant is usually portrayed as being localized on the surface of the folded polypeptide chain. Antigenic determinants fit into two distinct yet broad theoretical categories: sequential and conformational.[3]

Sequential Determinants

These are defined as those due to a particular sequence of amino acids or sugars in an unfolded or linear configuration. An antibody to one such sequence would be expected to react with all identical sequences.[3]

Conformational Determinants

These, on the other hand, result from a particular steric conformation of the antigenic macromolecule. They include amino acid residues which are brought into juxtaposition only in the folded protein.[4]

Of the whole determinant, only a small portion, usually the terminal unit in a sequential determinant, deserves the term "immunodominant." Such immunodominant portions contribute disproportionately to the binding energy in comparison to the area of the antibody-binding site which they fill.[5]

Blood Group Antibodies

All antibodies are immunoglobulins (Ig); they may be either IgG, IgM, IgA, or some combination of all three. For more detail about the structure and function of antibodies, see reference 6. Figure 1 is a schematic representation of an IgG molecule. An IgM molecule is

48

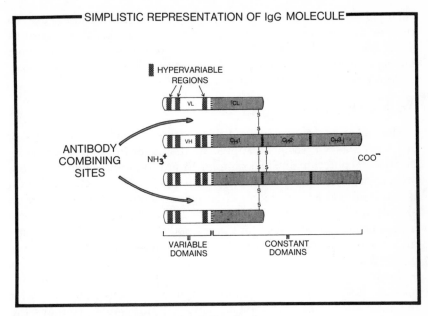

Fig 1.—Schematic representation of an IgG molecule.

a pentamer of five similar basic structures dispersed radially around a J chain 'clasp.' Ig molecules are flexible, but their 'stretch' or reach concerns the Stage of Coalescence, and will not be discussed here.

Antibody-Combining Sites

These sites are among the most remarkable recognition systems known. They are clefts at the NH_3^+-terminal end of the Fab subunits formed by spatial apposition of peptide loops containing the hypervariable regions. In general, the amino acid residues which define the clefts are derived predominantly from the heavy chains.[7] The exact shape and specificity or specificities are determined by only a few of the amino acids within or adjacent to the hypervariable regions; such amino acids may be termed "complementarity-determining".[5,8]

The sites occupy a shallow cleft or groove which may be as large as $1.5 \times 2 \times 1.2$ nm or as small as $1.6 \times 0.7 \times 0.6$ nm[7]; this is very small indeed compared with the overall size of any of the antibody molecules. IgG molecules have two combining sites, while IgM molecules have up to 10 available, depending upon the size of the determinant against which they are directed.

To put matters into perspective, imagine that a red cell has been enlarged to about the size of a page of this book. In relation to the red cell, the dimensions of an IgM molecule would be contained within a lower-case letter "o," and those of an IgG molecule within a comma. The size of the antigen receptor or the combining site of an antibody molecule would be completely invisible.[9]

Antibody Populations

The fact that monoclonal antibodies are nowadays the focus of attention makes it easier to appreciate that all ordinary immune antibodies are polyclonal. For example, in any one anti-D serum there are a number of discrete or subpopulations of anti-D. Each population is directed against a different D antigenic determinant, or differs in affinity for the determinant, or both. Incidentally, the fact that the measurements given above for the antibody-combining site were estimated using polyclonal antibodies makes it likely that they err on the high side.

The heterogeneity of antibody molecules to a defined determinant may be illustrated in part by using as a model an early paper showing the antibody response to the GIL hapten.[10] This hapten contains the amino acids glycine (G) and leucine (L) coupled to an isophthalic acid residue (I) which acts as a link. Figure 2 shows the steric outlines of the hapten and the four antibody populations fractionated from anti-GIL serum. Note that a straightforward anti-GIL population was not obtained. Instead, what the author has labeled anti-G, anti-IG, anti-IL, and anti-L were found; each varied both in concentration and affinity for antigen.

Crossreactivity

Another point to be emphasized is that, although the antigen: antibody reaction has a high degree of specificity, it is possible that two determinants belonging to two different antigens may be sufficiently similar in part of their structures, ie, have overlapping or shared structures, to lead to crossreactions with loosely binding antibody specifically raised against one or other of the antigens. Antibody-combining sites may also be polyfunctional.

Physicochemical Basis of Antigen-Antibody Binding

Adequate texts exist for those who wish to involve themselves in the intricacies of the thermodynamic and kinetic aspects of the antigen-

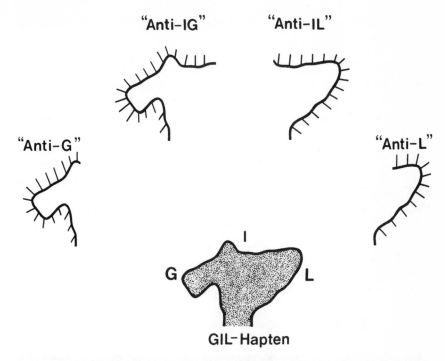

"Anti-IG"   "Anti-IL"

"Anti-G"   "Anti-L"

I

G   L

GIL-Hapten

Fig 2.—Steric outlines of GIL hapten and four antibodies produced in response to it (after Kreiter and Pressman[10]).

antibody reaction.[9,11-13] The author shall restrict himself to an outline based on the simplistic assumption that all antigenic determinants are identical and independent, and that one binding site of an IgG molecule or one or more sites of an IgM antibody molecule complexes with a determinant on one red cell membrane. The unattached site (IgG) or sites (IgM) are free to seek a determinant on another red cell (Stage of Coalescence).

Stereochemical Complementarity

Complementarity is often thought of as being solely structural—the "clenched fist" concept, where the clenched fist (antigen) fits into the concave palm (antibody) of the other hand. Undoubtedly the structure of the antigenic "probe" must fit into the antibody "cleft" if a stable complex is to be formed. But structure is the result of chemical composition. A close fit therefore depends upon complementarity of chemical groups on antigen and antibody.

51

Two stages are concerned in the formation of antigen-antibody complexes:

1. Structural complementarity. This step is highly specific.

2. Weak short-range intermolecular forces then come into play and keep antigen and antibody in apposition. Singly these forces are weak and nonspecific. However, when many bonds are formed simultaneously, they bring stability to the complex and may thus be considered to have some degree of specificity.

In Fig 3, it is clear that neither steric nor chemical fit alone is sufficient if bonding of antigen to antibody is to commence. In Fig 3(a) there is a good structural fit; furthermore, the chemical groupings are complementary. The result is that antibody will bind to antigen. In Fig 3(b), the structure of the antigenic receptor has altered, and steric fit is not possible, even though the chemical groupings are complementary. When the structures of the antigen receptor and the antibody combining site show a good structural fit but the chemical groupings result in forces which did not attract, and may even repel, there can be no effective combination or binding of antigen with antibody. (Fig 3(c)).

The physical coming together of antigen and antibody is essentially

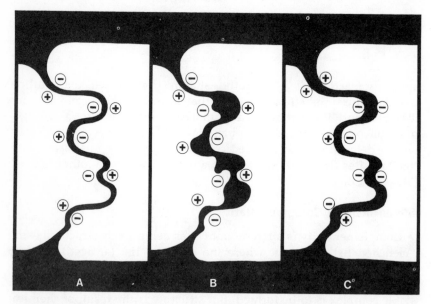

Fig 3.—Schematic representation of how steric fit and distribution of chemical groups are involved in antigen-antibody complex formation. Antigen is shown on the left; antibody on the right.

a process of random pairing of the two structures. It is entirely a matter of chance whether an antigenic determinant "bumps into" the binding site of an antibody molecule or vice-versa. If one bears in mind that antigenic determinants "have a three-dimensional electron-cloud shape, one can realize that, depending upon the direction from which the antibody molecule approaches," antibodies are confronted with very many different configurations even in a single determinant.[8]

The chance of an antibody molecule colliding with an appropriate antigenic receptor can be increased by some of the factors mentioned in Table 1, especially: (1) increase in the antibody concentration; and (2) numbers and accessibility of antigenic receptors.

Table 1—Some Variables Affecting the Formation of Specific Antigen:Antibody Complexes

Antigen	Antibody
Concentration	Concentration
Age of RBC	Ig classes, subclasses, types
Chemical nature	Heterogeneity:
Sites:	Number of concentration
Number	of discrete populations.
Accessibility	Mean and variance of
Arrangement	binding constants
Heterogeneity	

If an antigenic determinant does come into exactly the correct spatial relationship with a specific antibody-combining site as a result of Brownian motion or through artificial mechanical means such as agitation or centrifugation, the first stage of the reaction will begin.

Once antigen and antibody sites are in apposition, they are then held together by the weak, short-range chemical forces mentioned above. There is nothing special about these forces; they are essentially those which occur between any two unrelated macromolecules. Examples are hydrogen bonds, ionic bonds, polar interactions, hydrophobic effects, and van der Waals bonds. Each bond is the result of the combined, continuous action of bond-making and bond-breaking forces. The binding of antibody with antigen is, therefore, reversible.

The main point to be remembered is that, whatever the nature of the intermolecular forces involved, the greater the surface area of antibody site and antigen receptor in close proximity, the larger the number of bonds that can be formed. The larger the number of bonds, the greater the binding forces generated. Hence, the greater the "affinity" of antibody for antigen and the higher the value of K (see page XX).

As a result of the initial interaction of antibody with antigen, a time-dependent conformational change in both antibody and antigen contributes to the stabilization of the antigen-antibody complex.

Coulombic, Ionic, or Electrostatic Bonds

These are the result of attractive forces between a charged site on the antigenic receptor and an oppositely charged site in the antibody-combining cleft. They are primarily between the COO^- and the NH_3^+ groups on amino acids of antigen and antibody respectively,[13] and are inversely proportional to the square of the distance between the interacting groups.[13] The degree of ionization and the charge largely depend upon the pH of the medium (see pH, page 59).

Hydrogen Bonds

These bonds, formed between hydrophilic groups such as -OH, -NH-, and -CO-, are highly directional. They are also more specific and stronger than van der Waals bonds.

Hydrogen bonds are said by some[12,13] to contribute little to the stability of antigen:antibody complexes; others[14] disagree. This is not really a divergence of opinion: hydrogen bonds are probably not important when the antigen is protein, but they undoubtedly are when the determinant is carbohydrate. The stability of these bonds depends upon the presence of water molecules; their strength is augmented at low temperatures, ie, they are exothermic. The force of hydrogen bonds is inversely proportional to the sixth power of the distance between the atoms.[15]

van der Waals Attractive Forces

These are extremely short-range bonds which occur between all atoms and molecules if they are the correct distance apart; they result from the interaction of the electron clouds surrounding polar groups, and are inversely proportional to the seventh power of the interatomic distance.[13] The van der Waals radius is the distance from the centre of an atom to its steric outline; the correct distance for maximum attraction is the sum of these radii, which is in the region of 0.2-0.3 nm.[7] If the distance is greater than this, no attraction occurs.

London Repulsive Forces

Figure 4 illustrates these points, and also shows how a very slight decrease in intermolecular distance leads to strong repulsive forces. Repulsion is due to interpenetration of the electron fields, and is inversely proportional to the 12th power of the distance between the interacting groups,[13] ie, it is more sensitive to intermolecular distance than the forces of attraction. Such steric repulsive forces are as important as van der Waals attractive forces in antibody specificity.

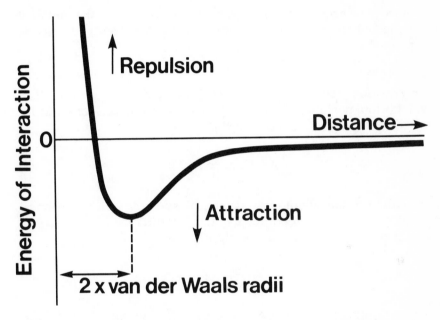

Fig 4.—Diagrammatic representation of effect of intermolecular distance on van der Waals forces.

Hydrophobic Effects

Interactions between apolar or hydrophobic particles in an aqueous environment are of particular importance in antigen-antibody binding.[12,13,16] Apolar groups, such as the side chains of valine, leucine, or phenylalanine,[8] have a strong tendency for self-association, with the result that solvent water is, figuratively, squeezed out. This expulsion of water (or tendency of water to bond to itself) decreases the distance between sites and thus greatly increases the attractive forces. These hydrophobic or dehydrating effects are principally side results of van der Waals-London interactions[12]; they may contribute "up to 50% of the strength of the antigen:antibody bond".[8]

The squeezed-out water molecules lead to a decrease in the free energy of the system (see page XX), because they assume a more random orientation when released. Hydrophobic effects are entropy-driven and endothermic; in contrast to hydrogen bonds the strength of interaction increases with temperature.[7]

Law of Mass Action

Since in principle all chemical reactions are reversible, the continual making and breaking of bonds between antigen and antibody may be expressed as:

$$Ag + Ab \rightleftharpoons AgAb \qquad (1)$$

This reaction proceeds in the forward and the reverse direction until an equilibrium position is reached[11]; it is governed by rate constants for association (k_a) and dissociation (k_d), thus:

$$Ag + Ab \underset{k_d}{\overset{k_a}{\rightleftharpoons}} AgAb \qquad (2)$$

According to the law of mass action, the speed at which a chemical reaction proceeds is proportional to the concentration of the reactants and their product. This may be expressed as:

$$\frac{[AbAg]}{[Ab][Ag]} = \frac{k_a}{k_d} = K_o \qquad (3)$$

where [Ab], [Ag], and [AbAg] represent the concentrations of antibody, antigen, and antibody-antigen complexes respectively. K_o is the average of the intrinsic association constants of the antibody populations under study; it is often referred to as the equilibrium constant.

Rates of Association and Dissociation

The bonds holding antigen and antibody in apposition dissociate and reassociate at different but progressively decreasing rates until an equilibrium is reached when the number of intermolecular bonds being formed per unit of time equals the number being broken. The reaction is thus in a state of relatively stable but dynamic equilibrium. The rate constants for association (k_a) and dissociation (k_d) can be determined experimentally, and an estimate then made of the order of magnitude of K_0.[17-19] These calculations of K_0 are based upon a number of assumptions,[11,18,19] one of which is that heterogeneity can be described by a normal Gaussian or Sips function. This may, in fact, not be so; distribution may be skewed or even bimodal.[20]

Antibody "Affinity"

Antibody affinity is a summation of the noncovalent intermolecular forces of attraction and repulsion involved.[13] Affinity is thus an expression of the primary binding energy of antibody-binding sites in a particular serum for the appropriate antigen receptors. It should not be confused with "avidity" which, although dependent on affinity, involves extrinsic factors.

Formation of an antigen-antibody complex causes a loss of free energy, because the molecules rearrange themselves in a condition of lower energy content. The "standard free energy" (ΔG^0) of a reaction places a figure on the amount of energy by which the complex is more stable than the individual isolated molecules; it is proportional to the logarithm of the average association constant, K, according to the equation

$$\Delta G^0 = -R \ T \ lnK$$

where R is the gas constant, T the absolute temperature in degrees Kelvin and ln is the natural logarithm.[7]

An estimate of affinity is given by the total strength of the bonds between antigen and antibody which, measured as the free energy change, has been found to lie between -10 and -14 kcal/mol for anti-c, -D, and -K1.[21] Since van der Waals forces contribute 1-2 kcal/mol per bond and ionic or hydrogen bonds 3-7 kcal/mol,[7] it follows that a number of bonds probably of different types are involved in cooperative interaction in any one antigen-antibody complex.

Mean Association Constant, K_0

A measure of the "goodness of fit" of antibody molecules for their corresponding antigenic determinants is given by the mean of the different association constants of all the discrete specific antibody populations in a serum. This value, K_0, falls within the range of 10^7-10^{10} 1/mol for anti-D and anti-K1.[11,21] Differences in estimates of K_0 are due primarily to heterogeneity in the rates of dissociation.[15,19] For example, a twofold difference between the highest and lowest values of k_a was seen with anti-D compared with a 15-fold difference for k_d.[19]

If the reasonable assumption is made that a certain minimum number of antibody molecules attached to each red cell is needed before the Stage of Coalescence can begin, then by rearranging equation (3) we have:

$$\frac{[AbAg]}{[Ag]} = K_0[Ab] \tag{4}$$

This shows that a critical threshold of $[AbAg]/[Ag]$ can be reached best when K_0 has a high value, ie, when the antibody has a high affinity for antigen. It follows that lower concentrations of antibody are needed to achieve this threshold when K_0 is high,[11] and vice versa.

From equation (4) it also follows that the power of detection of a test $[AbAg]$ will be highest when $[Ag]$ is lowest or, in more practical terms, when the ratio of serum to cells is as high as feasible. However, it has been estimated that this effect will not be observable when the value for K_0 is low.[22]

In routine work we use a serum:packed cells ratio of 100:1 or four volumes of serum to one volume of a 4% suspension of washed red cells. If dropper pipettes are used instead of semi-automatic pipettes with disposable tips, then the same pipette should be used for both serum and cells. In this way the wide fluctuations in serum:cells ratio reported by Beattie[23] can be avoided.

For maximum uptake of antibody as in manual fixation-elution tests, an excess of antigen is required. Equation (3) may once more be rearranged to demonstrate this:

$$\frac{[AbAg]}{[Ab]} = K_0[Ag] \tag{5}$$

Note that for routine antibody detection, this formula can be successfully applied only in such apparatus as the Auto-Analyzer.[24]

Effect of Environmental Factors on Antigen-Antibody Reactions

Temperature

As mentioned earlier, the reaction between antigen and antibody results in the release of free energy (ΔG^0). This energy may appear either as heat (exothermic reaction) or as a change in entropy (degree of randomness), or both. Exothermic reactions proceed further to com-

---

Table 2—Some Factors in the Reaction Environment that Influence the Demonstration of Hemagglutination

---

Ionic strength
pH
Temperature
Incubation time
Macromolecular media
Presence of complement
Centrifugation
Proteases

---

pletion at low temperatures, entropy-driven reactions at higher temperatures. Since hydrogen bonds are predominantly exothermic and associated with carbohydrate antigenic determinants, whereas hydrophobic effects are entropy-driven, it follows that "the determining factor which results in either 'warm' or 'cold' antibodies is the chemical nature of the antigen."[11]

In the case of "immune" antibodies so far studied, a rise in reaction temperature from 19-37 C has little effect on K_0 (about +25%),[18] but the rate of association is significantly increased (about $\times$ 2.5).[19] The rate of dissociation, wich is more heterogeneous, is slightly reduced at the colder temperature,[18,19] but this does not outweigh the greatly accelerated uptake of 'immune' antibody at 37 C.

pH

The isoelectric point (pI) of immunoglobulins—the critical pH at which positive and negative charges are in exact balance—covers a wide range and is indicative of heterogeneity. The subclasses of IgG show considerable variation, as shown in Table 3.

Table 3—IgG Subclasses; Frequencies and Isoelectric Ranges

	Subclass			
	IgG1	**IgG2**	**IgG3**	**IgG4**
Percent of total IgG[8]	65	23	8	4
Isoelectric range[25] (pH)	6.8-9.5	6.8-8.4	8.2-9	6

The only reference to the pI of blood group antibodies of which I am aware gives figures of 8.8 for anti-D, 8.9 for anti-LW, and 8.5 for the bulk IgG.[26] It is a great pity that more studies have not been done and related to IgG subclasses.

When the pH of the medium is lower, ie, more acid than the pI, protein molecules tend to be more positively charged. Theoretically, this could be an advantage, since red cells have a net negative charge which remains relatively unchanged between pH 7.0 and 6.0.[27] Antibody molecules, particularly the more basic IgG1 and IgG3, would therefore be more strongly attracted to them.

The rate of dissociation of anti-D is lowest and K_0 is highest when the pH is between 6.5 and 7.0.[28] Since about 95% of blood group antibodies so far tested belong to the IgG1 or IgG3 subclasses,[29] it seems likely that these data will hold true for other specificities.

Ionic Strength (I)

Whenever possible, the author has expressed lowered ionic strengths as a percentage of the isotonic value in order to permit comparison of data when different buffer systems with different degrees of ionization are used. Thus, in glycine-saline, an I of 0.03 is 80% less than isotonicity (I = 0.154); in glycine-PO_4 buffer, an I of 0.055 is 79% below isotonicity (I = 0.26).[30]

Hughes-Jones,[22,28] Masouredis,[30,31] and their co-workers independently showed the practical and theoretical advantages of a low ionic strength on the antigen-antibody reaction.

Increased Rate of Association

Hughes-Jones et al[28] found that for anti-D eluates there was a 1000-fold increase in the rate of association when the ionic strength of the reaction mixture was reduced by 82%. The rate of dissociation showed only a threefold fall.

Increased Uptake of Antibody

Atchley et al[30] found that 88% of the maximum uptake of anti-D was obtained in 10 minutes when the ionic strength of the reaction mixture was reduced 68%. This was a sixfold increase over antibody uptake at isotonicity. Figure 5 offers a comparison of the effect of low ionic and isotonic conditions on the rate of association and uptake of antibody. The time base, particularly under low ionic conditions, will almost certainly vary considerably from serum to serum because of the variables listed in Table 1.

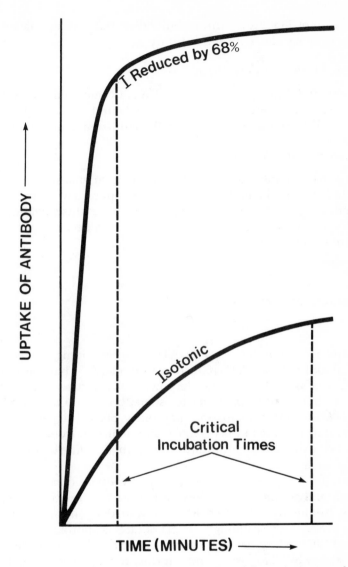

Fig 5.—Antibody uptake-time relationship of anti-D at different ionic strengths.

One most important advantage of using a low ionic strength during the Stage of Combination is that it provides conditions that favour uptake of low-affinity antibody. Hughes-Jones[22] has calculated that, for anti-D, changing from an isotonic to a low ionic milieu should enable 90-95% of antibody to become bound to the cells, an increase by a factor of 18 for low-affinity antibodies, but only by a factor of 1.2 for those molecules with high affinity.

Increased Uptake of Complement

A practical drawback is that complement components are taken up by the red cells at low ionic strength. This effect is maximal when I is reduced 80%, but disappears when the reduction is limited to 43%.[32]

Theoretical Considerations

It seems probable that in an isotonic medium ions such as Na^+ and Cl^- cluster around and partially neutralize oppositely charged groups on antigen and antibody. A reduction of I reduces this shielding effect, leading to an increase in electrostatic attraction between antigen and antibody and to a rise in k_a.[22,30]

Practical Considerations

LISS

Indirect antiglobulin tests (IDAT) using low-ionic strength solutions (LISS) with an 80% reduction in ionicity[33,34] have at last been recognized as enabling adequate powers of detection to be obtained in very short incubation times for some, but by no means all, antibodies. How short incubation may safely be will depend upon the period during which k_a is maximal; any reduction from the optimum will obviously lead to significantly less antibody being bound, particularly if K_0 is low.

Most IDAT (eg, reference 33) use equal volumes of cells suspended in LISS and serum to keep the I of the reaction mixture about 40% below isotonicity, at which level unwanted uptake of C' is not a major problem.[32,33] Although the pH of LISS is approximately 6.7, the serum:cells mixture has a pH about 0.2 below that of the serum, ie, approximately 7.2 for fresh serum; further reduction of the mixture pH to the theoretical optimum of 6.8-7.0[28] does not appear to have any practical advantage.

Polycations

Two recent reports[35,36] suggest that increased uptake of antibody can be obtained by IDAT if the I of the *reaction mixture* is reduced 80% by LISS in the presence of the polycations Polybrene™ or protamine sulphate. Problems due to increased uptake of C' can be minimized by using anti-IgG without anti-C'.

Bovine Serum Albumin (BSA)

Although the main effect of BSA is on the Stage of Coalescence, there is evidence that when BSA is present during the first stage of the indirect antiglobulin test (IDAT) the incubation period may be substantially reduced without any apparent loss in the power of detection of the test.[37-39] Since most lots of BSA have a low value of I (electrical conductivity equivalent to 0.09 mol/l NaCl, a 42% reduction from isotonicity, in recent lots I have used), and since BSA molecules bind anions such as Cl⁻ well, this serological effect of BSA may be due to a reduction in the shielding of charged groups, as mentioned above under Ionic Strength.

Proteases

The effects of proteases on haemagglutination are considered in a later chapter. This chapter points out only that one attribute, at least in the case of anti-D, is an increase in both k_a and K_0, and that the greatest increase occurs when the concentration of antibody is low.[40]

Summary

In vitro uptake of antibody by antigen, the Stage of Combination, depends upon two sets of factors, the one natural, the other environmental. Natural factors include the goodness of fit of antibody for antigen, the distribution of determinants and their chemical composition. Environmental factors are the relative concentrations of antigen and antibody, the pH and ionic strength of the reaction mixture, and the temperature and length of incubation. Over the first we have no control. Through the second the power of detection of our tests can be modified.

Acknowledgment

I thank Dr. J-P. Cartron of the C.N.T.S. Paris for his advice, and Dr. F. Ofosu, Mrs. Carol Laschinger, and Mrs. Rachel Berger of this laboratory for their helpful comments.

References

1. Wilson GS, Miles AA. The antigen-antibody reactions. In: Topley and Wilson's Principles of bacteriology and immunity. 3rd ed. London: Arnold, 1946:194.
2. Gill TJ III. The structural basis of immunogenicity and antigenic reactivity. In: Bell CA, ed. A seminar on antigens on blood cells and body fluids. Washington, DC: American Association of Blood Banks, 1980:25-32.3.
3. Sela M, Schechter B, Schechter I, Borek F. Antibodies to sequential and conformational determinants. Cold Spring Harbor Symp Quant Biol 1967;32:537-45.
4. Arnon R, Geiger B. Molecular basis of immunogenicity and antigenicity. In: Glynn LE, Steward MW, eds. Immunochemistry: an advanced textbook. Toronto: Wiley, 1977:307-63.
5. Williamson AR. Origin of antibody diversity. In: Glynn LE, Steward MW, eds. Immunochemistry: an advanced textbook. Toronto: Wiley, 1977:141-81.
6. Feinstein A and Beale D. Models of immunoglobulins and antigen-antibody complexes. In: Glynn LE, Steward MW, eds. Immunochemistry: an advanced textbook. Toronto: Wiley, 1977:263-306.
7. Watson JD. Molecular biology of the gene. 3rd ed. New York: Benjamin, 1979:85-111, 607.
8. Roitt IM. Essential immunology. 4th ed. Oxford: Blackwell Scientific Publications, 1980:1-42.
9. van Oss CJ. Precipitation and agglutination. 2nd ed. In: Rose NR, Milgrom F, van Oss CJ, eds. Principles of immunology. Toronto: MacMillan, 1979:80-106.
10. Kreiter VP, Pressman D. Antibodies to a hapten with two determinant groups. Immunochemistry 1964;1:151-63.
11. Hughes-Jones NC. Red cell antigens, antibodies and their interaction. In: Prankerd TAJ, Bellingham AJ, eds. Haemolytic anaemias. Clin Haematol 1975;4:29-43.
12. van Oss CJ, Absolom DR, Newmann AW. The antigen:antibody complex and erythrocyte destruction: physicochemical considerations. In: Sandler SG, Nusbacher J Schanfield MS, eds. Immunobiology of the erythrocyte: progress in clinical and biological research, vol 43. New York: Liss, 1980:157-69.
13. Steward MW. Affinity of the antibody-antigen reaction and its biological significance. In: Glynn LE, Steward MW, eds. Immunochemistry: an advanced textbook. Toronto: Wiley, 1977:233-62.
14. Cartron J-P. The ABO system. In: Salmon Ch, Cartron J-P,

Rougher Ph. The human blood groups: a series of lectures for graduate students. New York: Masson Inc., (in press).

15. Bach J-F. Antigen-antibody reactions. In: Bach J-F, ed. Immunology. Toronto: Wiley, 1978:248-60.

16. Singer SJ. Structure and function of antigen and antibody proteins. In: Neurath H, ed. The proteins: composition, structure, and function, vol III. London: Academic Press, 1965:269-357.

17. Hughes-Jones NC. Nature of the reaction between antigen and antibody. Br Med Bull 1963;19:171-7.

18. Hughes-Jones NC, Gardner B, Telford R. The kinetics of the reaction between the blood-group antibody anti-c and erythrocytes. Biochem J 1962;85:466-74.

19. Hughes-Jones NC, Gardner B, Telford R. Studies on the reaction between the blood-group antibody anti-D and erythrocytes. Biochem J 1963;88:435-40.

20. Werblin TP, and Siskind GW. Distribution of antibody affinities: technique of measurement. Immunochem 1972;9:987-1011.

21. Mollison PL. Blood transfusion in clinical medicine. 6th ed. Oxford: Blackwell Scientific Publications 1979:216, 217, 356.

22. Hughes-Jones NC, Polley MJ, Telford R, Gardner B, Kleinschmidt G. Optimal conditions for detecting blood group antibodies by the antiglobulin test. Vox Sang 1964;9:385-95.

23. Beattie KM. Control of the antigen-antibody ratio in antibody detection/compatibility tests. Transfusion 1980;20:277-84.

24. Rosenfield RE, Szymanski IO, Kochwa S. Immunochemical studies of the Rh system III. Quantitative hemagglutination that is relatively independent of source of Rh antigens and antibodies. Cold Spring Harbor Symp Quant Biol 1964;29:427-34.

25. Howard A and Virella G. The separation of pooled human IgG into fractions by isoelectric focusing, and their electrophoretic and immunological properties. In: Peeters H, ed. Proteins and related subjects, vol 17. Protides of biological fluids. Elmsford, NY: Pergamon Press, 1970:449-53.

26. Perrault R. "Cold" IgG autologous anti-LW. Vox Sang 1973;24:150-64.

27. Sachtelben P. The influence of antibodies on the electrophoretic mobility of red cells. In: Ambrose EJ, ed. Cell electrophoresis. London: J & A Churchill, 1965:100-14.

28. Hughes-Jones NC, Gardner B, Telford R. The effect of pH and ionic strength on the reaction between anti-D and erythrocytes. Immunology 1964;7:72-81.

29. Garratty G. Clinical significance of antibodies reacting optimally

at 37C. In: Butch S, ed. Clinically significant and insignificant antibodies. Washington, DC: American Association of Blood Banks, 1979:29-49.

30. Atchley WA, Bhagavan NV and Masouredis SP. Influence of ionic strength on the reaction between anti-D and D-positive red cells. J Immunol 1964;93:701-12.

31. Elliot M, Bossom E, Dupuy ME, Masouredis SP. Effects of ionic strength on the serologic behaviour of red cell isoantibodies. Vox Sang 1964;9:396-414.

32. Mollison PL, Polley MJ. Uptake of gamma globulin and complement by red cells exposed to serum at low ionic strength. Nature 1964;203:535-6.

33. Löw B, Messeter L. Antiglobulin test in low-ionic strength salt solution for rapid antibody screening and cross-matching. Vox Sang 1974;26:53-61.

34. Rouger Ph, Hertel F, Andreu G, Cartron J, Salmon Ch. Étude critique du test de Coombs à basses force ionique. Rev Fr Transfus Immunohematol 1980;XXIII:7-16.

35. Lalezari P, Jiang AF. The manual Polybrene test: a simple and rapid procedure for detection of red cell antibodies. Transfusion 1980;20:206-11.

36. Rosenfield RE, Shaikh SH, Innella F, Kaczera Z, Kochwa S. Augmentation of hemagglutination by low ionic conditions. Transfusion 1979;19:499-510.

37. Stroup M and MacIlroy M. Evaluation of the albumin antiglobulin technic in antibody detection. Transfusion 1965;5:184-91.

38. Cant B, Flamand C. The albumin antiglobulin test. Can J Med Technol 1967;29:101-2.

39. Wright J. Variations on a theme by Coombs. Can J Med Technol 1967;29:191-206.

40. Hughes-Jones NC, Gardner B, Telford R. The effect of ficin on the reaction between anti-D and red cells. Vox Sang 1964;9:175-82.

5

Red Blood Cell Agglutination: A Current Perspective

Edwin A. Steane, PhD

Introduction

WHEN APPARENTLY CONFLICTING HYPOTHESES ARISE covering any natural phenomenon, resolution is usually achieved as aspects of each hypothesis are integrated into a new whole. This seems to be an appropriate moment to begin such an integration relative to the subject of this paper, red blood cell agglutination.

Agglutination, and wherever used without qualification in this contribution, this word refers only to the clumping of erythrocytes by specific antibody, is generally considered to occur in two stages: sensitization, the attachment of antibody to the red blood cell surface, and agglutination proper, the crosslinking of the sensitized erythrocytes by antibody into visible aggregates. A distinct second stage can also occur, complement fixation, possibly leading to hemolysis, but this is not considered in this paper. These two stages occur at different rates, but once sufficient antibody has attached to initiate agglutination, proceed simultaneously to their individual equilibria. Dr. Moore[1] has discussed the first stage of agglutination in his companion paper in this volume. This paper will concentrate solely on the second stage.

Initially, certain historical aspects are outlined before proceeding to a discussion of some general concepts. An outline of the second stage of agglutination is then presented. It is not presumed that this paper presents a complete description of the phenomenon of agglutination, but rather an hypothesis upon which to base further experimentation.

Edwin A. Steane, PhD, Associate Professor of Clinical Pathology, Southwestern Medical School, The University of Texas Health Science Center at Dallas; Associate Director, Department of Hemotherapy, Parkland Memorial Hospital; Chief, Blood Bank, Veterans Administration Medical Center, Dallas, Texas

A Brief Historical Note

The Lattice or Crosslinking Hypothesis

An early idea of agglutination, noting the apparent requirement for the presence of electroytes, held that the attachment of antibody somehow resulted in nonspecific enhancement of an "agglutinating action of the electrolytes" (see Boyd[2(p343)]). With the arrival of the "lattice" theory,[3] most investigators have considered the reaction to be specific, in that the agglutinates are composed of erythrocytes held together by divalent antibody, one combining site of which is attached to one red blood cell, the other to a second. Although we now know that IgM is multivalent, this has not disturbed the general concept, in that one molecule of antibody links two erythrocytes, regardless of the number of antibody combining sites actually involved in attachment at each surface, because spatial relationships will not permit a single antibody molecule to interact with more than two erythrocytes. Even so, the problem of total specificity of the interaction cannot be considered resolved (see Boyd[2(p343, pp348-9)]), and the subject was still of sufficient concern to elicit a recent paper.[4] Under conditions of moderate antibody concentration, average antibody binding constant and high surface antigen site density, the agglutination of red blood cells can be considered specific.

Surface Charge and Hydrophobicity

Marrack[3] reviewed experiments conducted by Northrup and de Kruif[5] with bacteria, noting that agglutination occurred in the presence of electrolytes below a critical surface potential of -15 mV, that is, if the potential was between zero and -15 mV. Marrack[3] also recognized the hydrophilic/hydrophobic state as important in suspension stability. His observations are sufficiently pertinent to later discussions that direct quotation of two short sections is appropriate. In discussing the effect of high salt concentration on bacterial agglutination he comments[3(p134)]: "It must be inferred that, when the salt concentration is raised, a change takes place on the surface of the bacteria, leading to a reduction of the mutual attraction of the bacteria, or an increased attraction for water, a change from a hydrophobe to a hydrophil state." This concept, essentially that of interfacial tension, will recur throughout the description of agglutination advanced in this paper. Later in his monograph Marrack[3(p137)] makes the following important statement: "If, however, the antigens are not fully sensitized the change from hydrophil to hydrophobe is less complete, and the critical potential for agglutination is lower." In other words, the attachment of antibody increases surface hydrophobicity. If surface hydrophobicity is increased, the critical potential above which agglutination will not occur is less negative. (The concept of greater or lesser, higher or lower, for quantities preceded by a negative sign always presents a problem, and in 1977 gave rise to a series of letters in *Transfusion* under the heading "Zeta potential in hemagglutination."[6] Although the author favors the Mollison approach as stated in his letter,[6] an attempt is made to clarify the meaning in each instance in this paper.) This idea appears to be still valid. As with the first sentence quoted, this second sentence will form the basis for the extended description of surface phenomena, and the interrelationship of interfacial tension and electrical repulsion in particular, presented later.

Pollack's Zeta Potential Theory

Pollack[7] and Pollack and associates[8] presented a theory of agglutination which became popularly known as the zeta potential theory. Briefly, the argument advanced was that an intercellular distance was maintained between erythrocytes due to the repulsion generated by the negatively charged red blood cell surface. IgG molecules were unable to bridge the intercellular gap, whereas IgM molecules, being larger, could bring about crosslinking. This hypothesis provided a ready explanation for the difference between the agglutinating potential of incomplete versus complete antibodies. If the zeta potential of the erythrocyte was measured as more negative than -23 mV, it was shown that agglutination would not occur, even with IgM antibodies. At minus seven mV red blood cell suspension stability was compromised. Optimal zeta potential for agglutination by IgM antibodies was found to be -18 mV; for IgG antibodies minus eight mV. That proteolytic enzymes decreased surface charge, and thus zeta potential, was proposed as the explanation for their serological action. Albumin, known to promote the hemagglutination of Rh positive erythrocytes by incomplete anti-D, was thought to bring about agglutination by increasing the dielectric constant of the suspending solution, thereby decreasing the erythrocytic zeta potential (see next section).

Pollack and his associates[8] recognized the importance of interfacial tension, but tended to minimize its influence. Likewise, they were under the misapprehension that IgM molecules could span a distance some four times greater than IgG molecules. Repulsion due to the negatively charged surface-associated sialic acid moieties remains an important concept, but it now appears that it can be counterbalanced by the cohesive forces of interfacial tension more easily than Pollack and his coworkers supposed.

In the early 1960s, at the time that the zeta potential model for the second stage of agglutination outlined above was developed, others[9,10] were demonstrating that surface charge and agglutination were probably not that closely related. In fact, Haydon[11] commented: "Specific agglutination effects are likely to be governed by the actual number and character of the surface ionogenic groups rather than by the net electrophoretic charge. . . ." With regard to the agglutination of Rh positive erythrocytes by IgG anti-D, the phenomenon of particular interest to Pollack's group, the 1973 paper by Stratton et al[12] indicated the non-viability of a charge-zeta potential model. That agglutination by IgG molecules in saline was not only possible, but dependent upon the number of antigenic sites was demonstrated by Leikola and Pasenen[13] in 1970.

The Importance of Water and Interfacial Tension

From their studies of the agglutination of neuraminidase-treated red blood cells, Greenwalt and Steane[14] proposed that the degree of hydration at the erythrocyte surface had a controlling influence upon the second stage of the agglutination reaction, an idea that had occurred to Hummel (see Gold and Peacock[15(p219)]). Recent studies by Masouredis et al[16] have ascribed the enhancement of agglutination by proteolytic enzymes to changes in the biophysical properties of the red blood cell membrane, and Steane and Gregory[17] have presented preliminary evidence that the major change is probably in interfacial tension.

It is not the purpose of this paper to review the past literature concerning erythrocyte agglutination, and readers who would like to familiarize themselves with the problems involved are referred to recent reviews by this author,[18-21] which have appended references to much of the original literature. This paper will present the author's current understanding of the complex nature of the agglutination reaction, and this brief historical note is intended to outline the development of specific ideas which are integrated into a single conceptual framework here. A brief but tantalizing abstract by Reckel and Pollack[22] indicates that Pollack and his co-workers have probably reached similar conclusions.

General Concepts

The Hydrophobic Effect and the Dynamic Flux of Cellular Membranes

In the first edition of his book, *The Hydrophobic Effect*, Tanford[23(pvii)] wrote as the first sentence of his preface: "The hydrophobic effect is perhaps the most important single factor in the organization of the constituent molecules of living matter into complex structural entities such as cell membranes and organelles."

This "effect," common to our everyday experience, but still imperfectly understood, forms the backbone of our understanding of cell membrane structure and interaction. It is general knowledge that cell membranes are composed of bilipid layers. It is recognized by many that such bilipid layers form ideal "barriers" which demarcate the cell from its environment, and compartmentalize the cell contents. Formation of these barriers is understood by most at a basic level: the lipid molecules are amphipathic, and the polar "heads" wish to remain in contact with the aqueous environment, whereas the hydrocarbon "tails," disliking water, form bilayers through headgroup contact with water as the fatty acid chains "hide" within the bilayer. It must be understood that membranes form because of the hydrophobic effect, and at the same time cellular hydrophobic effects are the result of the specific composition of the membrane.

It is also important that this concept be extended. Lipid molecules in an aqueous environment, even in a membrane, are not static. A membrane, once built of lipid "bricks" is not like a wall of house bricks, but a dynamic interface. Lipid molecules can move relatively freely in the plane of the membrane, and can leave the surface. Other lipids can be incorporated into the membrane by adsorption from the plasma, a fact well known to immunohematologists through study of the Lewis blood group system, but still somehow considered an isolated instance, a special case, rather than an example of the dynamic flux of living matter. Throughout this paper, the lack of "permanence" of the interacting molecules must be understood. Whatever affects one macromolecule is likely to affect neighboring macromolecules. Every interaction must be considered with respect to this structural dynamism.

As an example, let us consider some of the possible changes that occur as cholesterol is added to or removed from the erythrocyte membrane. In the first place, this addition or removal is affected by temperature: but not only is the degree of addition or removal so affected, the changes that this addition or removal bring about are also

71

temperature sensitive. A change in cholesterol content alters the "fluidity" of the membrane, the degree to which it is rigid or pliable. It also alters the hydrophobicity of the membrane surface, and the degree to which this alteration occurs will depend upon whether the cholesterol exchanges with another lipid molecule or whether it is inserted or removed without changing the remainder of the membrane lipid constitution. If an exchange does occur, which lipids are exchanged will also determine the change in hydrophobicity. Further, other membrane components within the membrane may undergo rearrangement or repositioning with respect to a change in the cholesterol to other lipids ratio.

Each of these changes can affect agglutination, as we shall note later, but deciding which is the most significant change, or to what degree each change affects the final result observed, is what makes an investigation of the phenomena associated with living matter so complex. One can make the following analogy: it is relatively easy to toss a ball from one hand to the other, and two balls can be mastered with little effort, but three balls requires diligence, patience, practice, determination and, perhaps, a certain talent. It is the willingness to recognize the dynamic state of the interacting macromolecules, to become a biochemical juggler, which permits the beginning of conceptual understanding. When one adds to this the individuality of these macromolecules in any given case (see Levin[24]), despite the general nature and the "blindness" of the natural forces involved, it is little wonder that many despair. Concrete descriptions of biological phenomena are unlikely until we possess far more knowledge than at present. It is impossible to overstress the importance of this concept, and it is for this reason that it is discussed at such length.

Membrane Structure with Specific Reference to Erythrocyte Membrane Composition and Topography

Although originally the erythrocyte membrane was thought to represent a prototype for study, we now realize that is is unique, and spectrin, the protein which forms the basis of the red blood cell membrane cytoskeleton, has not been found in other cells. However, certain concepts have been derived from the study of erythrocyte membranes which seem to be generally applicable. First, the membrane is asymmetric with respect to lipid composition. In the erythrocyte, phosphatidylcholine and sphingomyelin are more abundant in the external half of the bilipid layer, whereas phosphatidylserine and phosphatidylethanolamine are found in greater concentration in the cytoplasmic face. Second, carbohydrate is confined to the outside of the plasma membrane, and is linked to protein or lipid as glycoprotein or glycolipid; there are no free oligosaccharide molecules in membranes. Third, proteins are also asymmetrically distributed. Either the protein is an intrinsic or integral protein, which indicates that it is embedded in and probably always traverses the bilipid layer, or it is an extrinsic or peripheral protein, in which case it is a surface protein, loosely attached by noncovalent interaction to either the inner or outer face, and readily removed by relatively mild changes in environmental conditions, such as an alteration of ionic strength. Integral proteins that have been well studied have three domains. These are the external domain, characterized by attached oligosaccharide sidechains, a membrane domain, composed of hydrophobic amino acids, representing that portion of polypeptide actually in contact with the lipid bilayer, and an internal or cytoplasmic domain, in which hydrophilic amino acids predominate, and to which no carbohydrate is attached. More complex proteins which traverse the membrane more than once are visualized; similarly, complexity through subunit interaction is certainly possible. Peripheral proteins at the outside surface are not necessarily synthesized by the cell, in fact, this is somewhat unlikely. Erythrocytes have many peripheral proteins at the inside surface, few, if any, at the external surface. Susan Steane[25] has published an excellent review of erythrocyte membrane composition with the knowledge needs of the serologist in mind.

We now recognize that in erythrocytes much of the surface area is lipid and glycolipid, and that protein molecules are relatively well dispersed within the bilayer matrix. These proteins also protrude to a significant distance above the bilipid layer outer face, and a picture of frequent isolated mountains towering above a grassy plain is probably not too far from reality. For a more detailed description of current thoughts concerning red blood cell membrane topography see Steane.[21]

Water Structure as the Basis for Cell Surface Interfacial Tension

In discussing the hydrophobic effect, and its ordering force with respect to cell membranes, it is important to consider water itself. Water has a strong tendency to self-associate. This is consistent with experience. Water falling through air tends to form drops; to minimize its surface area. This self-association is the basis for the phenomenon we know as surface tension. When in contact with a hydrocarbon, such as benzene, this tendency to self-association is also evident, as is a similar tendency of the hydrocarbon. We all know that oil and water "do not mix."

What happens in any particular mixture of hydrophobic and hydrophilic molecules is dependent upon their relative concentrations. If we shake the correct proportions of vinegar and oil, for instance, we obtain salad dressing, an emulsion which separates relatively slowly into its component parts. This process of separation can be slowed further by adding emulsifiers, often natural phosopholipids, which result in the formation of more stable lipid micelles provided, once again, the proportions are correct. Micelles, which are either globular balls of lipid with their polar headgroups in contact with the aqueous environment and their apolar hydrocarbon chains buried inside, or small cell-like bilipid layer structures, have a critical size. Above this size they become unstable. Mammalian cell membranes are complex structures far greater in size than the largest natural micelles in which the tendency to instability is substantially overcome by the incorporation of proteins, both as integral parts of the membrane structure and as an underlying cytoskeleton.

A bilipid layer possesses a surface tension at the water-lipid interface due to the properties of the water and lipid discussed above. In the classic paper describing their bilipid layer proposal for membrane structure, Danielli and Davson[26] recognized that the surface tension of cell membranes was too low to be consistent with a surface composed of polar lipid headgroups. In a companion paper, Danielli and Harvey[27] reported results with mackerel egg oil and cells which indicated that the cell surface possessed a remarkably decreased interfacial tension over that expected, and that this decrease was due to a protein component of the cell membrane. Although the Danielli and Davson explanation of a layer of protein adsorbed to the surface proved incorrect, their thesis remains intact: the surface tension of cells is decreased by other macromolecules associated with the lipid bilayer, components which we now recognize to be glycoproteins and glycolipids. Red blood cells, because of their low interfacial tension, have little tendency to aggregate spontaneously, and suspension stability is maintained under these conditions by electrostatic repulsion. Should there be an increase in interfacial tension there would be a dramatic shift in the energy balance affecting cell-cell interaction.

Electrostatic Repulsion and Zeta Potential

Electrostatic repulsion is generated by glycolipids and glycoproteins which bear the negatively-charged carbohydrate, N-acetylneuraminic acid. The nature of electrostatic repulsion is known to nearly everyone from everyday experience. Most have experienced the force of attraction and repulsion generated by magnets, and are aware of the increase in force as the magnetic poles are brought closer together. We can assume a similar increase in force as two red blood cells approach closely, but must carefully consider the likely consequences in terms of intermolecular distances basing our hypothesis on what we know of erythrocyte surface topography.

Charged groups attract counter ions in solutions of electrolytes such as sodium chloride. Some of these ions travel with the cell as a kinetic unit. The density of the counterion layer is a function of the density of the charged groups at the cell surface, and the ionic strength and dielectric constant of the bulk medium. As the distance from the surface increases, there is a decrease in attractive force such that the cloud of ions "thins out," eventually reaching the same concentration as the ions in the bulk medium. At that distance from the cell within which volume the cloud of ions is part of the cell kinetic unit, a potential drop relative to the cell surface can be theorized. This potential is known as the zeta potential, and is inversely related to the ionic strength and dielectric constant of the bulk medium. Zeta potential is usually inferred from measurements of cell mobility in an electric field.

Summary

It is on these general concepts that the remainder of this paper rests: that the membrane, an asymmetric construct of proteins, glycoproteins, lipids and glycolipids, is in dynamic equilibrium, both with regard to the molecules of which it is composed and the external and internal environment; that water has a high surface tension; that the normal red blood cell has a relatively low interfacial tension in aqueous electrolyte solution; and that the erythrocyte has a net negative surface charge, mainly as a result of the sialic acid-bearing glycoproteins we call the glycophorins. The description of the second stage of the agglutination reaction which follows recognizes that each antibody that binds to a surface antigen, each modification of technique that we make, changes the relationship of charge to surface tension, and perhaps the relative position, even three-dimensional structure, of the component molecules. Each individual antigen-antibody interaction must be examined from this perspective. There can be no simple, all-inclusive model which applies in every case, although there are some applicable general principles. It is these general principles that the next section attempts to describe.

The Second Stage of Agglutination

In the preceding section, four general concepts have been discussed: membrane composition and the dynamic state of living matter; erythrocyte surface topography; interfacial tension; and erythrocyte net negative surface charge and zeta potential. It will be useful to consider a few further topics before proceeding to the main discussion.

Attractive and Repulsive Forces

Attractive and repulsive forces in aqueous media are of four types: ionic (or electrostatic), hydrogen bond, van der Waals and hydrophobic. Extended discussion of these forces is inappropriate for this paper. A few important points will be emphasized.

Ionic forces between biological macromolecules result from the interaction of charged amino acid side chains (see Steane[25] for a more detailed discussion) and the negatively charged carbohydrate N-acetylneuraminic acid. Do not misinterpret this sentence to indicate that amino acid side chains interact with sialic acid-bearing proteins or lipids; this is not what it means. Wherever charged macromolecules come into close approximation there will be an an attraction or repulsion; the *sources* of the charges are the amino acid side chains and sialic acid. In each case the resultant attraction or repulsion depends upon the composition of the macromolecules, the distance between them, the ionic strength of the surrounding medium (and its dielectric constant), and the pH. pH has no effect, at least within normal physiological limits, on strongly-charged acid (such as sialic acid) or basic (such as lysine) molecules, but the charge of molecules such as histidine is altered by an alteration in pH.

Hydrogen bonding occurs between many carbohydrates and amino acids. Once again, this sentence should not be misinterpreted. Hydrogen bonding can occur *between* carbohydrates; it also occurs between amino acids, both *within* a single polypeptide chain (hydrogen bonding is the most important determinant of the initial folding of a protein) and *between* different polypeptide chains, as in the interaction between heavy and heavy, and heavy and light chains in immunoglobulins. It *can* also occur between carbohydrates and amino acids. Hydrogen bonding can be regarded, physicochemically, as a special instance of the generalized phenomenon of van der Waals interactions. These interactions are of three basic types: induced dipole–induced dipole, permanent dipole–permanent dipole, and permanent dipole–induced dipole. A dipole is an area of opposite charge *within* an atom or molecule. All atoms have constantly changing instantaneous dipoles as the electrons move in their orbits around the nucleus. These interactions can be attractive or repulsive. Hydrogen bonding is an example of a permanent dipole-permanent dipole interaction. For a more detailed discussion of van der Waals interactions see Nir.[28]

Similarly, hydrophobic interactions can logically be argued to result from van der Waals interactions, and are again a special case. Hydrophobic interactions result from the hydrogen-bonding properties of water, and are thus an extension of the discussion of the previous paragraph. It can be concluded, therefore, that there are but two sets of basic intermolecular forces, electrostatic and van der Waals. We continue to discuss interactions in terms of hydrogen bonding and hydrophobic forces because these are convenient descriptive terms which permit "visualization" of the interaction, but the underlying foundation for all these weak interactions is the electrical nature of matter.

The Electrical Double Layer

Any charged macromolecule in an electrolyte-water solution will be surrounded by a cloud of ions. This concept has already been discussed as the basis for the zeta potential of the red blood cell. As macromolecules surrounded by this ionic cloud approach closely, the ionic clouds interact. This double layer interaction results in a free energy change dependent upon the degree of overlapping of the double layers. In general, this free energy change between identical surfaces is unfavorable, and the interaction is manifested as a repulsion.

The Hydration Repulsion

All polar charged and noncharged macromolecules in water solution will be surrounded by a thin layer of tightly bound water molecules. If two such macromolecules are to interact, work is required to remove this hydration shell in order to permit the interacting surfaces to approach closely. This required work is also manifested as a repulsion.

The Effect of Ionic Strength

As the concentration of electrolyte in a given solution increases, the ionic double layer around charged macromolecules is compressed in thickness. Consequently, charged surfaces can approach more closely before experiencing a double layer interaction. In general, we can state that increasing the ionic strength enhances net attraction when the double layer forces are repulsive and decreases it when the double layer forces are attractive.

Since this is an important point, elaboration by example is probably advisable. Consider an hypothetical antigen and antibody such that there is a net negative charge on the antigen and a net positive charge on the antibody. Antigen and antibody would be attracted to each other and this attraction would be enhanced when the double layer interaction occurs through sufficiently close approach. Increasing the ionic strength would decrease this attraction; decreasing the ionic strength would increase the attraction. If we are considering the approach of two erythrocytes, the situation is reversed. Here, the double layer interaction results in repulsion. Increasing the ionic strength leads to a decrease in repulsion; decreasing the ionic strength to an increase in repulsion.

The Effect of Salts

"Salting-out" of proteins is familar to many immunohematologists, since ammonium sulfate added to serum results in the precipitation of immunoglobulins. This can be understood as an interfacial tension effect, but the underlying explanation is again the result of van der Waals interactions and the special properties of water. For an excellent discussion, see Srinivasan and Ruckenstein.[29] In general, solutes "fit" into defined cavities within the solvent. When the solvent is water there are constraints imposed by the water molecules such that if these constraints are intensified the solute cannot be contained and precipitates. Table 1 gives some surface tensions for salt solutions. An increase in surface tension indicates that the inclusion of the salt has caused the free water molecules (those not intimately associated with the salt molecules) to bond together more strongly. This provides less "room" for other solutes, which can be displaced from solution. On

Table 1.—Surface Tension of Aqueous Salt Solutions at 25 C*

Salt	Concentration	Surface Tension (dynes/cm)
Amonium sulfate	3M	78.4
Sodium chloride	3M	76.9
(Water)		72.0
Tetraethyl ammonium chloride	1M	57.0
Guanidinium chloride	4M	51.0

*Adapted from Lewin[30] and Srinivasan and Ruckenstein.[29]

the other hand, those salts which decrease surface tension permit greater solubility for other solutes.

The Effect of Organic Solvents

Adding organic solvents to aqueous solutions of macromolecules has two major effects. First, they lower the dielectric constant of the bulk medium. Table 2 presents some dielectric constant figures for

Table 2.—Surface Tension of Organic Solvents*

Solvent	Dielectric Constant	Surface Tension (dynes / cm)
(Water)	78.3	72.0
Ethylene glycol	40.7	46.7
Dimethyl sulfoxide	46.7	43.5
Dimethyl formamide	36.7	36.8†
n-Propanol	20.3	23.7

*Adapted from Srinivasan and Ruckenstein.[29]
†At 20 C, all others at 25 C.

selected solvents. Electrostatic double layer interactions are enhanced by a decrease in dielectric constant. At the same time, surface charge is likely to be reduced, since dissociation is decreased and charge pairing and partial neutralization are increased. Therefore, the net effect may be minimal. One can understand this at a basic level by recognizing that all charge effects increase as dielectric constant decreases, since charge is more fully expressed (less dissipated) under these conditions. Although the basic phenomenon may be described in these simple terms, the net result is not simple, as can be seen from the above, because the same change in the environment can cause different effects among the complex macromolecular entities involved. It is the resultant new balance which determines the final observed effect of adding an organic solvent.

Second, organic solvents substantially reduce van der Waals attractions. This is because they break down the tendency of the water to form instantaneous ice-like structures because of their decreased tendency to participate in hydrogen bonding. As always, there are differences depending upon the polar or nonpolar nature of other macromolecules in solution in the balance of attractive and repulsive forces, so the change expected following the addition of an organic solvent cannot always be predicted by a general statement. However, one can predict that the addition of an organic solvent will decrease the attraction between molecules held together by van der Waals attractive forces, but if electrostatic attraction is also involved, one may have to change the pH in order to decrease the intensity of this interaction to achieve separation. This is the basis for the elution procedure described by van Oss et al.[31]

Agglutination: the Balance of Cohesive and Repulsive Forces

Theories of agglutination to date can be reduced to three basic models[15]: the charge repulsion-zeta potential model; the hydration shell model; and the steric hindrance model. It is proposed that all three models can be combined given the following assumptions: (1) there is a repulsion between red blood cells in electrolyte solution which normally maintains dispersion of the erythrocytes; (b) this repulsion can be overcome by sufficient crosslinks forged by antibody molecules, or if other forces push the red blood cells together; (c) one such force pushing erythrocytes together is the natural cohesive force of van der Waals attraction, manifested as interfacial tension; (d) interfacial tension is altered by several manipulations employed by serologists, and also by the attachment of antibody (as is electrostatic and hydration repulsion); (e) crosslinking will still depend upon where the antigen is situated within the glycocalyx, and this may change as conditions within the microenvironment change, and upon the number of antigenic sites available for antibody attachment.

We have already discussed charge repulsion effects, which, in electrolyte solution, are mainly the result of the double layer interaction. We can use the symbol R_C to denote this repulsion. There is also a hydration repulsion, as outlined above, the result of the polar nature of the red blood cell surface, which we can designate R_H. The overall repulsion, which we can simply call R, is the sum of $R_C + R_H$. Similarly, we can denote the natural cohesive forces, due mainly to the van der Waals attractions manifested as interfacial tension, as A. If A is greater than R, the red blood cells will spontaneously aggregate; if R is greater than A, the erythrocytes will approach to some defined distance determined by the magnitude of R and A. Since for erythrocytes in physiological saline, R is greater than A, we can write the equation:

$$\text{degree of separation} = R - A.$$

Neuraminidase specifically removes N-acetylneuraminic acid from the erythrocyte surface eventually decreasing the zeta potential to zero, yet neuraminidase-treated erythrocytes do not spontaneously aggregate in saline. Why is this? Remember that Danielli and Davson[26] noted that cell membranes had a lower interfacial tension than expected due to protein, actually glycoprotein, incorporated into the membrane, and the explanation becomes clear. An erythrocyte from which all the sialic acid has been removed still has a low interfacial tension, and has no inclination towards aggregation. However, crosslinking by antibodies should be facilitated, because the effect of electrostatic repulsion has been somewhat decreased. Note that it has been replaced by a hydration repulsion, since the removal of a sialic acid molecule results in the exposure of an underlying galactose or galactosamine molecule, to which N-acetylneuraminic acid molecules are always attached. Figure 1 presents some data relating the degree of increase in agglutination of group A_1 erythrocytes by IgG anti-A following neuraminidase treatment. There is an immediate effect as charge decreases, but this is not sustained. This is because there is a decrease in the double layer

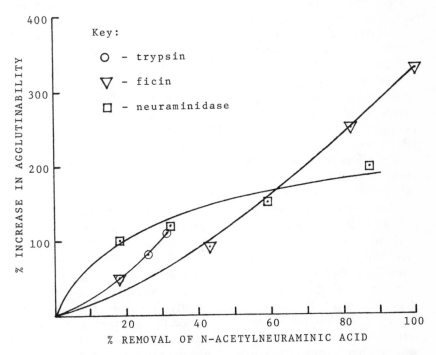

Fig 1.—The increase in agglutinability of neuraminidase-, trypsin-, and ficin-treated group A_1 red blood cells by anti-A. Percent agglutinability is expressed as the increase over the agglutination (10%) of untreated erythrocytes by a standard dose of antiserum. Percent sialic acid released is expressed as a function of the maximal release by ficin treatment. (Data redrawn from Steane.[32])

interaction as the sialic acid at the red blood cell periphery is removed. Removal of more deeply buried sialic acid has little effect, and hydration repulsion becomes the major determinant of cell separation. The degree to which hydration repulsion generated by glycoprotein maintains cell separation can be discerned by comparing the neuraminidase curve to the ficin curve, in which much of the hydration repulsion has been abolished and interfacial tension effects predominate. Cleaving of proteins from the red blood cell surface decreases charge and increases interfacial tension. One is removing the Danielli-Davson protein coat, exposing the underlying bilipid layer. A, in our equation above, is increased. The marked effect that this has can be observed, particularly when the trypsin curve in Fig 1 is compared to the ficin curve. Ficin is much more efficient at hydrolyzing protein than trypsin, and the ficin-treated erythrocyte is essentially shorn of all surface protein, whereas a considerable protein coat remains even after maximal trysin treatment.

Again, ficin-treated erythrocytes do not spontaneously aggregate in saline. Interfacial tension, though altered, is not changed sufficiently to overcome the remaining repulsion. This repulsion is due to the hydration repulsion generated by the polar nature of the lipid headgroups and the repulsion generated by the negative charge of the phosphate group of the phosphatidylcholine and small amounts of sialic acid attached to glycosphingolipids. The *balance* of repulsion versus attraction is altered in the suspensions of neuraminidase- and ficin-treated red blood cells, and Fig 1 demonstrates the degree to which these two forces affect agglutination by anti-A. Charge repulsion is a relatively minor opponent of crosslinking by specific antibody; hydration repulsion a rather constant underlying feature of the interaction. Changes in interfacial tension, if you like, removal of a good measure of the hydration repulsion, play a dominant role, and can markedly facilitate crosslinking and agglutination by antibody.

There is a theoretical steric repulsion associated with cell surface glycoprotein which is the result of the free energy change due to the mutually excluded volumes of the polymer chains. Greig and Jones[32] have analyzed this and shown that the repulsion, as expected, is dependent upon the amount and density of glycoprotein at the cell surface. Additionally, the force calculated is very large relative to the force arising from the overlap of the electrical double layers. This could add another term to the equation presented above, or it could be a component of the hydration repulsion term. In any case, since it is proportional to the glycoprotein content, as is the hydration repulsion, treatment of erythrocytes with proteolytic enzymes will markedly decrease this repulsion. This additional complexity does not change the general nature of the arguments presented above, but is included for the sake of completeness, and will not be considered further.

It should be apparent by now that any change which occurs by natural means, such as the binding of antibody, or which we impose, by manipulation of technique, is likely to result in many possible effects, some of which may be counterbalancing. Whether agglutination occurs depends upon the *net* balance of forces acting at reaction equilibrium. The remaining sections of this manuscript will describe this balance and its alteration under those conditions commonly used in the serological laboratory.

Normal Ionic Conditions

Under normal ionic conditions, that is, the conditions that apply for "saline agglutination," the balance of opposing forces is such that red blood cell separation is maintained in the absence of specific antibody uptake. Note that this is true for nearly all conditions we shall discuss. It is not the intent of this statement to characterize suspension stability as different under normal ionic conditions. Suspension stability effects are observed when the attractive forces of antigen-antibody interaction are superimposed. The distance to which the erythrocytes approach is largely determined by the double layer interaction due to the charged outer surface. When antibody attaches, this repulsion is altered. The degree to which it is altered is mainly dependent upon the number of antibody molecules which attach, although some consideration to where the antibody attaches is required. Unfortunately, our knowledge base is insufficient for most blood group antigens for other than speculation.

Sachtleben and Ruhenstroth-Bauer[9] and Sachtleben[34] demonstrated the effect of antibody uptake on electrophoretic mobility. Saturating erythrocytes with anti-A caused a 30% decrease in mobility, whereas fully anti-D coated red blood cells did not alter in mobility. Washing the anti-D coated cells and reacting them with an antiglobulin serum produced a decrease in mobility. Anti-M and anti-N, on the other hand, agglutinated prior to any measurable change in mobility, but the addition of increasing amounts of antibody resulted in a precipitous drop. These workers interpret their data, probably correctly, as evidence that there is no direct correlation between charge and agglutination.

Why do these different antibodies cause different effects? We know that the site density of the A antigen is enormous in comparison to the density of antigens of most other blood group systems; it is therefore not surprising that some effect of protein adsorption is noted. D antigenic sites are far less numerous; the amount of protein specifically adsorbed to a maximally coated D-positive erythrocyte would only be 2-4% that attached to a maximally coated group A red blood cell. It is significant to note that agglutination induced by anti-A begins before a measurable change in electrophoretic mobility occurs, but that with saline-active anti-D, no change can be detected in mobility even when agglutination is maximum. IgM molecules, therefore, can span the separation distance of saline-suspended red blood cells and bring about agglutination. Whether or not they do so will almost certainly depend upon antigen site density and the binding constant of the specific antibody. The separation distance is apparently of no consequence regardless of where the antigen resides within the erythrocyte glycocalyx.

However, IgG anti-A can cause agglutination, and the degree to which it does so is directly correlated to antigenic site density.[35] Other IgG antibodies can cause agglutination also: as shown by Leikola[36] and Leikola and Pasanen,[13] it is the antigen site density which is the determinant of whether agglutination will occur, not the class of the antibody. Since this still implies that impediments to close approach must be overcome, many remain cloudy as to the objection to a simple charge repulsion explanation. Were charge repulsion the explanation, agglutination would occur readily following neuraminidase treatment, and it does not, particularly with antibodies specific for antigens of low site density; repulsion is due to other than electrostatic double layer interaction.

At high site density, many molecules attach. This very attachment leads to a decrease in electrostatic repulsion, probably due to shielding of charged groups by adsorbed protein. There is also a decrease in the hydration repulsion. Not only are erythrocytes less repelled, there is an actual increase in attraction due to the change in interfacial tension, and they agglutinate. When insufficient molecules attach the balance of forces is not altered to the extent needed to permit agglutination. Repulsive forces generated by sialic acid molecules are able to maintain suspension stability and erythrocyte separation under natural conditions, not under the driving force of attraction provided by antigen-antibody interaction. Under these circumstances the red blood cells will approach more closely, but still not agglutinate. This is because their closeness of approach is counterbalanced by the hydration repulsion, and this repulsive force can only be overcome by a change in interfacial tension or some other manipulation. IgM molecules will support agglutination under normal ionic conditions; IgG molecules will not unless a sufficiently large number attach to overcome hydration repulsion, or unless other means, for example centrifugation, are imposed to force, and hold, the erythrocytes close enough to permit a sufficient number of antibody crosslinks to form which can withstand the reimposition of repulsion when the artificial means of bringing about close approach is removed. If there are not sufficient crosslinks formed, agglutination will still not occur unless the biophysical properties of the red blood cell membrane are also changed.

Agglutination by antiglobulin reagents, although possible under normal ionic strength conditions, is still subject to some repulsion between the erythrocyte surfaces, as is agglutination by IgM. Again, the number of crosslinks formed and the binding constant of the antibody for its antigen will determine the degree of resultant agglutination. In the case of antiglobulin reagents, there are two binding constants to consider, both the antibody for its antigen, and the antiglobulin molecule for the antibody. It is not surprising that antiglobulin reactions can also be favored if repulsion effects, once again mainly due to the hydration repulsion, are diminished.

Increased Ionic Strength

When ionic strength is increased red blood cells can approach more closely before experiencing repulsion due to the double layer interaction. However, attraction of antigen for antibody, whether mainly electrostatic or van der Waals in nature, is at the same time decreased. In the resulting changed balance, only antigens of high site density are likely to benefit from decreased double layer interaction repulsion, since decreased antibody uptake is not as significant at high density. ABO blood group system antibodies result in somewhat increased agglutination at high ionic strength, as might be expected.

Not enough careful measurements for the majority of blood group antibody specificities have been made to ensure that antibody uptake is always decreased under high ionic strength conditions. Decreased van der Waals and electrostatic interactions may also be but part of the reason for decreased uptake. Alterations in the three dimensional shape of the antigen and antibody molecules due to altered intramolecular forces is certainly a possibility.

Decreased Ionic Strength

Decreasing the concentration of electrolyte should have the opposite effects to those described in the paragraph above. Erythrocytes cannot approach as closely before experiencing the double layer interaction, but antigen-antibody interaction will be favored. However, even though the cells cannot approach as closely as under normal ionic conditions, the repulsion is likely to be decreased since the ionic cloud is not as concentrated. The net effect is that although antibody uptake is increased, there is not likely to be a significant enhancement of agglutination. In fact, one could suspect that agglutination by anti-A (or any other IgG antibody able to cause direct agglutination) might be somewhat decreased over that obtained under normal ionic conditions if the serum antibody concentration is low.

There is another facet of the reaction under low ionic conditions; the alteration of interfacial tension due to nonspecific adsorption of protein to the red blood cell surface. This adsorption is favored for similar reasons to those which result in an increase in specific antibody uptake. When protein is adsorbed there is a change in surface hydrophobicity. The surfaces interacting in the protein-erythrocyte surface attraction are mainly hydrophilic; the net result is an "apparent surface" somewhat less hydrophilic than before the addition of the protein coating. There is considerable experimental evidence to support this mechanistic explanation, but much work remains to be done. There can be some alteration of electrostatic repulsion simply by adsorption of positively charged protein molecules to the negatively charged glycoproteins and glycolipids. The net result of this protein adsorption at very low ionic strength is the spontaneous aggregation of the suspended erythrocytes due to altered interfacial tension (increased attraction) and decreased electrostatic repulsion. This leads to the false positive agglutination familiar to immunohematologists if an attempt is made to increase the benefit of decreased ionic conditions by lowering the electrolyte concentration too far.

Albumin

Some controversy still exists concerning the action of albumin in the hemagglutination reaction. In general, there is little effect on antibody uptake (the first stage of the reaction) even at relatively high concentrations of polymerized albumin.[37] There is a definite effect of albumin, particularly polymerized albumin, on the second stage, that is, agglutination.[38] This effect was hypothesized by Pollack et al[8] to be due to a decreased electrophoretic mobility (and thus zeta potential) because albumin increased the dielectric constant of the bulk medium. Brooks et al[39] showed, to the contrary, that whatever other effects albumin might have, it does not decrease zeta potential. If one accepts that zeta potential is not the determinant of closeness of approach, and therefore of agglutination, then an alternative explanation for the undoubted effect of albumin can be advanced.

Albumin, at normal concentration but under low ionic strength conditions, binds to the outer face of the phospholipid bilayer.[40] When the concentration of albumin is increased at normal ionic strength, a similar binding can be supposed, the mass action equilibrium being shifted by increased concentration rather than an increase in nonspecific attractive forces. Interfacial tension will change, favoring agglutination. Polymers can be expected to increase this change in interfacial tension simply because they "cover" a larger area of the phospholipid interface. Polymer bridging[39] between erythrocytes may play some role, but this author suspects that interfacial tension has already been so markedly altered at the concentrations required for spontaneous aggregation that separating an attraction of the erythrocytes mediated by polymer bridging from aggregation resulting from a shift in the cohesive-repulsive energy balance will be difficult. Certainly, other colloids, notably dextran,[41] can go from aggregation to repulsion as the size of the polymer is increased. This fits an alteration in energy balance better than a bridging hypothesis, since one must recognize that total covering of the surface results in two surfaces totally covered with hydrophilic material, and one would expect that hydration repulsion will then again dominate the energy balance.

Other Colloids

Little needs be said about the effect of other colloids. Their effect will relate to their ability to alter the cohesion-repulsion balance through their effect on electrostatic repuslion, hydration repulsion and interfacial tension. One would expect that interfacial tension effects will predominate at moderate concentrations and, as with albumin, hydration repulsion effects will rule at high concentration, if the macromolecule binds to the red blood cell surface.

For the sake of completeness, one must consider the effect that albumin and other colloids might have on the bulk medium. Any molecule capable of forming hydrogen bonds with water molecules will tend to compete with any other macromolecule for its share of the available water molecules. This is similar to the effect earlier called salting out. Polyethylene glycol, for example, is an excellent protein precipitant. Most serologists are aware of the marked aggregating effect of high colloid concentrations on erythrocyte suspensions. This effect is best visualized as a change in interfacial tension favoring attractive over repulsive forces.

Proteolytic Enzymes

An alteration in the cohesive forces promoting attraction has already been postulated as the major effect of removing the glycoproteins that are responsible for the lower interfacial tension of the erythrocyte; removing them increases the tendency to aggregation promoted by the interfacial tension generated at the outer face of the bilipid layer. Adding the attraction produced by specific antigen-antibody interaction results in agglutination.

Since agglutination is favored following proteolysis, red blood cells can form aggregates provided the antigen site density is sufficiently high to support crosslinking. There will still be a remaining hydration repulsion, already discussed, so that if the antigenic site is so situated that very close approach is required at very low antigen site density, agglutination may be possible by the antiglobulin method when it is not easily achieved by the enzyme technique, simply because this hydration repulsion is less effective at the increased erythrocyte separation required for agglutination by antiglobulin molecules.

Cationic Polyelectrolytes

The positively charged polymers Polybrene[R] and protamine sulfate aggregate erythrocytes through complex coacervation (see van Oss et al[42]). Complex coacervation is the aggregation of macromolecules of opposite charge in the presence of water. It should be noted that this phenomenon is not yet completely understood, and although oppositely charged macromolecules are required, the effect is not mediated through charge alone. When the negative charge of red blood cells is decreased by neuraminidase action or proteolysis, complex coacervation does not occur, and the erythrocytes do not aggregate. Although coacervates formed in the presence of serum are easily reversed by the addition of sodium citrate, coacervates formed in saline solution in the absence of protein are not easily neutralized. The exact mechanism by which complex coacervation occurs in a mixture of an erythrocyte suspension and a positively charged macromolecule is not known, and worthy of considerable study.

Coacervates form most readily at low ionic strength, and since this also promotes antigen-antibody interaction, there is obviously a great potential for a simple serological test, as realized by Rosenfield et al[43] and Lalezari and Jiang.[44] The method has been used in the AutoAnalyzer[R] for a longer period.[45] "Subtracting-out" any residual aggregation is relatively easy in the AutoAnalyzer,[R] but is difficult by eye, a fact which has delayed acceptance of the manual low ionic polycation test.

For the serologist, this test clearly demonstrates the principles of agglutination. If the forces of repulsion can be overcome, and the red blood cells brought close enough, agglutination will occur, and one can almost say regardless of the specificity and class of the antibody. Once the coacervation is reversed, whether or not the agglutinates remain stable depends upon whether the number of antigen-antibody bonds formed can withstand the repulsion which is reimposed. This depends both upon their number, which in turn depends upon antigen site density and antibody concentration, and the affinity constant of the particular antigen and antibody combination. A further consideration applies, namely, where the antigen is within the glycocalyx. Surprisingly, it may not be the most deeply buried antigens which result in the strongest repulsion when sodium citrate or dilution reverse the aggregation brought about by the polycation, but this subject is too complex for this paper. Interested readers are referred to Watt and Ward[46] for a short discussion of the long range effect of the intermolecular forces discussed in this paper. This facet of antigen-antibody interaction has been exploited by Lalezari,[47] but its potential for increasing our understanding of blood group antigen-antibody interaction is only now beginning to be realized.

That steric hindrance is not a significant bar to agglutination is revealed by this technique. Not only do nearly all antibodies react regardless of specificity, the glycocalyx must be quite compressed during the aggregation phase, and none of it is removed, as has been used to explain the success of proteolytic enzymes inpromoting agglutination.[12] One major exception seems to be anti-Kell. A possible explanation for this is that the polycations bind to the Kell antigen-bearing macromolecule, but this seems unlikely, since it appears to be low ionic conditions which decrease the reactivity of anti-Kell, since even in the polycation test the antiglobulin test is weaker than under normal ionic conditions. It appears likely that a three dimensional change in antigen is likely at low ionic strength, perhaps indicating an important role for electrostatic interaction in defining the shape of the Kell antigen. We shall have to wait until more is known concerning the biochemistry of the Kell system before we can fully explain the lack of agglutination by antibodies of this specificity.

Membrane Flexibility and Aldehyde Fixation

If agglutination can only be supported by sufficient antibody bridges, this would imply that erythrocyte surfaces in apposition should be distorted when agglutinated if antigen site density is low. Electron microscopic analysis appears to confirm that they are. Fixation of erythrocyte membranes by formaldehyde and glutaraldehyde results in a marked decrease in agglutination, even if the red blood cells have been subjected to prior treatment by proteolytic enzymes. Progressive treatment eventually results in the erythrocytes becoming inagglutinable. Carbohydrate antigens appear to be able to fix their corresponding specific antibody regardless of the degree of fixation, but the binding to other antigens such as Rh, which appear to contain no carbohydrate, is diminished and with progressive treatment abolished. This latter is probably due to distortion of the three-dimensional shape of the antigenic molecules, but it could be due to a change in charge and van der Waals interactions between antigen and antibody following the crosslinking of proteins in the membrane by the fixative. For the decrease in the second stage of agglutination, which occurs even though antibody is well fixed, the decrease in membrane flexibility seems sufficient as an explanation. It is possible that the binding of the fixative changes the repulsion due to electrostatic or hydration mechanisms but this seems unlikely (see Vassar et al[48]). A decrease in the already low interfacial tension can be discounted.

Aldehyde-fixed erythrocytes can be agglutinated by lectins if the agglutinates are not subjected to shear forces; that is, if the degree of agglutination is read from the settling pattern.[49] Marquardt and Gordon[49] also demonstrated that fixed erythrocytes will form mixed agglutinates with unfixed erythrocytes in suspensions subjected to moderate shear forces, which they ascribe to the flexibility of the unfixed membrane accommodating the rigid fixed membrane. The added complexity of shear forces on agglutination is not considered in this paper. Greig and Brooks[50,51] have proposed three classes of agglutination: static, type I and type II; the latter two are shear-force induced. This added complexity will need to be integrated into our overall scheme of agglutination when it has been studied more intensively.

Cholesterol in Erythrocyte Membranes as an Example of the Complexity of the Agglutination Phenomenon

Alderson and Green[52] demonstrated changes in red blood cell agglutination by phytohemagglutinin when cholesterol was added to, or removed from, the membrane. Addition of cholesterol increased agglutination at the same dose of lectin; cholesterol depletion decreased agglutination. Although these authors considered antigen mobility, which would be increased by cholesterol enrichment, as a possible explanation, this will be discounted here as a negligible factor in the agglutination of adult human erythrocytes (see Schekman and Singer,[53] Masouredis et al[16]).

Shinitzky and Souroujon[54] have demonstrated a change in the expression of the D antigen following cholesterol enrichment or depletion. At a cholesterol to phospholipid ratio (C/PL) of 1.55, twice as much antibody was bound as at a C/PL of 0.65. Unmodified erythrocytes have a C/PL of 0.95. Under similar conditions group A_1 red blood cells bound 20% more antibody at the highest C/PL compared to the lowest. Agglutination by anti-A was considerably enhanced (titer 560) at the highest C/PL compared to the lowest (titer 140). This lipid fluidity-modulated change in antigenic expression has been termed "passive modulation" by Shinitzky.[55] A theoretical discussion of these changes relative to interfacial tension has been presented by Gerson.[56] Plapp and his associates[57] have proposed that the difference between Rh-positive and Rh-negative erythrocytes is the modulation of a similarly-sized Rh gene-specified protein by other membrane components. This protein, when isolated from Rh-negative erythrocyte membranes, would inhibit the interaction of anti-D with Rh-positive cells in a hemagglutinating system.

Although many more experiments are needed, it appears that we can say that in general agglutination will be enhanced by the incorporation of cholesterol into the membrane. This can occur through at least three possible mechanisms: (1) cholesterol increases the fluidity of the membrane, an effect we can consider the opposite of aldehyde fixation; (2) cholesterol causes the modulation of antigens such that they are more exposed at the membrane surface, they are "raised up"; (3) interfacial tension is increased, and the erythrocytes are more predisposed to agglutinate when reacted with specific antibody. Modulation of antigen will also decrease the distance that antibody must span if the antigen is forced up within the membrane, but modulation in the opposite direction is certainly a possibility. Each of these mechanisms can operate individually, in opposition, or in concert in any given instance. It is this type of multiple effect which we must study and understand before we can completely comprehend and separate out the relative importance of the individual parts within the complex whole. Although not yet demonstrated, a possible change in the three-dimensional configuration of noncarbohydrate antigens should be considered as an added complexity as studies of membrane lipid-enriched or -depleted red blood cell agglutination are expanded.

Spiculation: the Discocyte-Echinocyte Equilibrium

Whenever a double layer interaction occurs, the repulsion generated can often be overcome by decreasing the area of the surfaces in contact. A flexible erythrocyte membrane can form protrusions when washed free of plasma and suspended in physiological saline. The transformation from a relatively smooth biconcave disc to a somewhat swollen "sea urchin"-like structure covered with spicules has been termed the discocyte-echinocyte transformation by Bessis.[59] Such protrusions are able to penetrate the electrostatic repulsion barrier with relative ease. The degree to which this is of relevance in agglutination remains to be precisely determined, but van Oss et al[42] think that it is extremely important. References to the original papers and further discussion can be found in a recent review.[20] It is mentioned here to illustrate the myriad changes which must be considered in discussing this complex phenomenon. For this author, it is of relatively little importance, since he knows of no antibody specificities which agglutinate consistently when diluted in saline which do not agglutinate when serum is present. In fact, a high concentration of serum is more likely to promote agglutination than the production of spiculation by its removal. However, Marikovsky et al[60] have published evidence that the echinocytic transformation of erythrocytes by lysolecithin increases the rate of their agglutination by soybean lectin and of their aggregation by poly-L-lysine. Whether these increases are the result of spiculation, or changes in hydrophobicity and receptor modulation such as discussed in the preceding section pertaining to cholesterol, remains to be determined with certainty. It does appear that *fimbriae* (see Watt and Ward[46]) promote adherence of bacteria to eukaryotic cells, so the importance of cellular protrusions within the overall energy balance should not be dismissed out of hand.

Concluding Remarks

In this paper, the concept of cohesive forces, mainly van der Waals interactions manifested as interfacial tension, versus repulsive forces, mainly the double layer interaction of similarly charged macromolecules in electrolyte solution, and the hydration repulsion generated by surface hydrophilic macromolecules, has been explored as the mechanistic underpinning influencing erythrocyte agglutination.

An attempt has been made to keep the description of the inter-molecular forces simple, and no effort has been made to discuss the mathematics and other considerations which underlie the descriptions presented. Interested readers are referred to the papers by Dolowy and associates[61,62] if they wish to begin further exploration of the concepts expounded upon in this contribution. In general, it is held that hydra-tion repulsion is the major repulsive force preventing the close approach of sensitized erythrocytes. A description of the generation of this repulsion by hydrophilic glycoproteins has been given. Removal of these glycoproteins converts the erythrocyte surface into a more hydrophobic structure, promoting close approach. This concept of interfacial tension change is fundamental to the description of aggluti-nation proposed. Electrostatic repulsion is considered to play little role in preventing agglutination by specific antibody. Antibody binding also decreases repulsion and promotes agglutination through its alteration of surface effects as well as through specific bridging. It is because of these factors that antigen site density assumes such critical importance. As Marrack[3] realized so long ago, the degree to which repulsion can maintain separation is in part dependent upon the degree to which antibody adsorption can convert the cell surface from its normal hydrophilic to a more hydrophobic state. Many of the technical manipulations invented by serologists have attempted to achieve the same end.

It is hoped that many careful measurements in well-designed and controlled experiments will be carried out over the next years to con-firm or refute the overwhelming importance ascribed to interfacial tension effects. In addition, immunohematologists would do well to look to the literature of bacterial adherence and phagocytosis, cellular recognition and response modulation, and all aspects of protein-protein interaction to follow the struggles of fellow scientists with the same basic set of problems.

Acknowledgments

I would like to thank my wife, Susan, for acting as a sounding-board during the writing of this manuscript. Any ideas which appear to be expressed with clarity are in no small part due to her persistence. My secretary, Mrs. Phyllis Kitterman, has once again turned out a model typescript. Only those who have seen the handwritten copy and the continuing revisions can truly appreciate her herosim.

References

1. Moore BPL. Antibody uptake: the first stage of the hemagglutination reaction. In: Bell CA, ed. Antigen-antibody reactions revisited. Washington, DC: American Association of Blood Banks, 1982.
2. Boyd, WC. Fundamentals of Immunology. 4th ed. New York: Interscience, 1966.
3. Marrack JR. The chemistry of antigens and antibodies. London: HM Stationery Office, 1938.
4. Romano EL, Mollison PL. Mechanism of red cell agglutination by IgG antibodies. Vox Sang 1973;25:28-31.
5. Northrup JH, De Kruif PH. The stability of bacterial suspensions. III. Agglutination in the presence of proteins, normal serum, and immune serum. J Gen Physiol 1922;4:655-67.
6. Schorr JB; Issitt PD, Issitt CH; Pollack W; Mollison PL. Zeta potential in agglutination, letters. Transfusion 1977;17:288-9.
7. Pollack W. Some physicochemical aspects of hemagglutination. Am NY Acad Sci 1965;127:892-900.
8. Pollack W, Hager HJ, Reckel R, Toren DA, Singher HO. A study of the forces involved in the second stage of hemagglutination. Transfusion 1965;5:158-83.
9. Sachtleben P, Ruhenstroth-Bauer G. Agglutination and the electrical surface potential of red blood cells. Nature 1961;192:982-3.
10. Brody OV, Oncley JL. Effect of erythrocyte net charge upon agglutination and rouleaux formation. In: Sawyer PN, ed. Biophysical mechanisms in vascular hemostasis and intravascular thrombosis. New York: Appleton-Century-Crofts, 1965:239-42.
11. Haydon DA. The surface charge of cells and some other small particles as indicated by electrophoresis. II. The interpretation of the electrophoretic charge. Biochim Biophys Acta 1961;50:457-62.
12. Stratton F, Rawlinson VI, Gunson HH, Phillips PK. The role of zeta potential in Rh agglutination. Vox Sang 1973;24:273-9.
13. Leikola J, Pasanen VJ. Influence of antigen receptor density on agglutination of red blood cells. Int Arch Allergy 1970;39:352-60.
14. Steane EA, Greenwalt TJ. Red cell agglutination. Experimental evidence suggesting an important role for vicinal water. In: Mohn JF, Plunkett RW, Cunningham RK, Lambert RM, eds. Human blood groups. Basel: Karger, 1977:36-43.
15. Gold ER, Peacock DB. Antigen-antibody reactions. In: Gold ER, Peacock DB, eds. Basic immunology. Baltimore: Williams and Wilkins, 1970.

16. Masouredis SP, Sudora EJ, Victoria EJ. Immunological and electron microscopic analysis of IgG anti-D saline agglutination of neuraminidase- and protease-modified red cells. J Lab Clin Med 1977;90:929-48.

17. Steane EA, Gregory KJ. A simple method for estimating red blood cell surface hydrophobicity, abstract. Transfusion 1981;21:602.

18. Steane EA. The physical chemistry of hemagglutination. In: Walker RH, ed. A seminar on polymorphisms in human blood. Washington, DC: American Association of Blood Banks, 1975: 105-127.

19. Steane EA. The interaction of antibodies with red cell surface antigens: kinetics, noncovalent bonding, and hemagglutination. In: Dawson RB, ed. Blood bank immunology. Washington, DC: American Association of Blood Banks, 1977: 61-86.

20. Steane EA, Greenwalt TJ. Erythrocyte agglutination. In: Sandler SG, Nusbacher J, Schanfield MS, eds. Immunobiology of the erythrocyte. New York, Liss, 1980, pp 171-88.

21. Steane EA. Erythrocyte agglutination. Red cell membrane topography and the role of interfacial tension. Clin Lab Med 1982;2:155-67.

22. Reckel R, Pollack W. The importance of interfacial free energy and hemagglutination, abstract. Abstracts, Intl Soc Blood Transf, Montreal, 1980:30.

23. Tanford C. The hydrophobic effect. 2nd ed. New York: Wiley, 1980.

24. Levin R. Biology is not postage stamp collecting. Science 1982; 216:718-20.

25. Steane SM. Basic membrane biochemistry and its relationship to blood group serology. In: Bell CA, ed. A seminar on antigens on blood cells and body fluids. Washington, DC: American Association of Blood Banks, 1980:1-24.

26. Danielli JF, Davson H. A contribution to the theory of permeability of thin films. J Cell Comp Physiol 1934;5:495-508.

27. Danielli JF, Harvey EN. The tension at the surface of mackerel egg oil, with remarks on the nature of the cell surface. J Cell Comp Physiol 1934;5:483-94.

28. Nir S. Van der Waals interactions between surfaces of biological interest. Prog Surface Sci 1976;8:1-58.

29. Srinivasan R, Ruckenstein E. Role of physical forces in hydrophobic interaction chromatography. Sep Purif M 1980;9:267-370.

30. Lewin S. Displacement of water and its control of biochemical reactions. London: Academic Press, 1974.

31. van Oss CJ, Beckers D, Engelfriet CP, Absolom DR, Neumann AW.

Elution of blood group antibodies from red cells. Vox Sang 1981; 40:367-71.

32. Steane EA. Thermodynamic studies of erythrocyte antigen-antibody interaction and the modulation of this phenomenon by partial enzymatic digestion of the cell membrane, PhD dissertation. The George Washington University, Washington, DC, 1974.

33. Greig RG, Jones MN. The possible role of steric forces in cellular cohesion. J Theor Biol 1976;63:405-19.

34. Sachtleben P. The influence of antibodies on the electrophoretic mobility of red blood cells. In: Ambrose EJ, ed. Cell electrophoresis. Boston: Little, Brown, 1965:100-114.

35. Cartron JP, Gerbal A, Hughes-Jones NC, Salmon C. 'Weak A' phenotypes. Relationship between red cell agglutinability and antigen site density. Immunology 1974;27:723-7.

36. Leikola J. Studies on the nature of incomplete anti-Rh antibodies. Int Arch Allergy 1967;32:474-81.

37. Leikola J, Perkins HA. Red cell antibodies and low ionic strength: a study with enzyme-linked antiglobulin test. Transfusion 1980; 20:224-8.

38. Reckel RP, Harris J. The unique characteristics of covalently polymerized bovine serum albumin solutions when used as antibody detection media. Transfusion 1978;18:397-406.

39. Brooks DE, Seaman GVF. The effect of neutral polymers on the electrokinetic potential of cells and other charged particles. I. Models for the zeta potential increase. J Colloid Interface Sci 1973; 43:670-86.

40. Donath E, Steidel R. Electrostatic and structural properties of the surface of human erythrocytes. Acta Biol Med Germ 1980; 39:207-15.

41. Brooks DE. Effect of macromolecules on aggregation of erythrocytes. In: Mohn JF, Plunkett RW, Cunningham RK, Lambert RM, eds. Human blood groups. Basel: Karger, 1977:27-35.

42. Van Oss CJ, Mohn JF, Cunningham RK. Influence on various physiocochemical factors on hemagglutination. Vox Sang 1978; 34:351-61.

43. Rosenfield RE, Shaikh SH, Innella F, Kaczera Z, Kochwa S. Augmentation of hemagglutination by low ionic conditions. Transfusion 1979; 19:499-510.

44. Lalezari P, Jiang AF. The manual Polybrene test: a simple and rapid procedure for detection of red cell antibodies. Transfusion 1980;20:206-11.

45. Lalezari P. A new method for detection of red cell antibodies. Transfusion 1968;8:372-80.
46. Watt PJ, Ward ME. Adherence of *Neisseria gonorrhoeae* and other *Neisseria* species to mammalian cells. In: Beachey EH, ed. Bacterial adherence. London: Chapman and Hall, 1980:251-88.
47. Lalezari P, Berens JA. Specificity and cross reactivity of cell-bound antibodies. Implications in autoimmune hemolytic diseases. In: Mohn JF, Plunkett RW, Cunningham RK, Lambert RM, eds. Human blood groups. Basel: S. Karger, 1977:44-55.
48. Vassar PS, Hards JM, Brooks DE, Hagenberger B, Seaman GVF. Physicochemical effects of aldehydes on the human erythrocyte. J Cell Biol 1972;53:808-18.
49. Marquardt MD, Gordon JA. Glutaraldehyde fixation and the mechanism of erythrocyte agglutination by concanavalin A and soybean agglutinin. Exp Cell Res 1975;91:310-16.
50. Greig RG, Brooks DE. Shear-induced concanavalin A agglutination of human erythrocytes. Nature 1979;282:738-9.
51. Greig RG, Brooks DE. Enhanced concanavalin A agglutination of trypsinized erythrocytes is due to a specific class of aggregation. Biophys Biochim Acta 1981;641:410-15.
52. Alderson JCE, Green C. Lectin-induced cell agglutination and membrane cholesterol levels. Exp Cell Res 1978;114:475-9.
53. Schekman R, Singer SJ. Clustering and endocytosis of membrane receptors can be induced in mature erythrocytes of neonatal but not adult humans. Proc Natl Acad Sci USA 1976;73:4075-9.
54. Shinitzky M, Souroujon M. Passive modulation of blood-group antigens. Proc Natl Acad Sci USA 1979;76:4438-40.
55. Shinitzky M. The concept of passive modulation of membrane responses. In: deLisi C, Blumenthal R, eds. Physical chemical aspects of cell surface events in cellular regulation. Amsterdam: Elsevier North-Holland, 1979:173-81.
56. Gerson DF. Interfacial free energies and the control of the positioning and aggregation of membrane proteins. Biophys J 1982; 37:145-7.
57. Plapp FV, Evans JP, Tilzer LT, Chiga M. Quantitation of Rh_0 (D) antigen on the inner and outer membrane surface of Rh positive and negative erythrocytes, abstract. Abstracts, Intl Soc Blood Transf, Montreal, 1980:264.
58. Evans JP, Plapp FV, Tilzer LL, Beck M, Chiga M. Rh_0 (D) and LW antigen content of Rh null erythrocytes, abstract. Transfusion 1980; 20:618.

59. Bessis M. Red cell shapes. An illustrated classification and its rationale. In: Bessis M, Weed RI, Leblond PF, eds. Red cell shape. New York: Springer, 1973:1-24.

60. Marikovsky Y, Brown CS, Weistein RS, Wartis HH. Effects of lysolecithin on the surface properties of human erythrocytes. Exp Cell Res 1976;98:313.

61. Dolowy K, Holly FJ. Contribution of interfacial tension changes during cellular interaction to the energy balance. J Theor Biol 1978; 75:373-80.

62. Dolowy K, Godlewski Z. Computation of the erythrocyte cell membrane parameters from electrophoretical and biochemical data: Stern-like electrochemical mode of the cell membrane. J Theor Biol 1980;84:709-23.

6

Potentiators of Agglutination

John Case, FIMLS

Introduction

THE PHENOMENON OF HEMAGGLUTINATION provides the most convenient means of studying reactions between red cell surface antigens and their corresponding antibodies. In its simplest form the test requires only the barest minimum of equipment. It may be performed on a microscope slide, on some other suitable flat or concave surface, in a test tube, a capillary, or in any container having sufficient capacity to accommodate the reaction mixture comprising serum and a suspension of red cells.

Whether working with unknown cells and a serum containing an antibody of known specificity, or with an unknown serum and red cells possessing a known antigen, the test result is clearcut. Agglutination of the test red cells yields readily-observable evidence that a specific antigen-antibody reaction has taken place, while the absence of agglutination should testify to the contrary. Such, at any rate, was the premise on which were based the conclusions reached by Landsteiner when he discovered the ABO groups.[1] The same simple test procedure enabled Landsteiner and Levine to characterize the M, N and P_1 antigens,[2,3] and also served Landsteiner and Wiener in studying the Rh factor.[4] The method used to study the immune response of the animals injected with rhesus monkey red cells, and to determine the frequencies of Rh-positive and Rh-negative among human bloods, was a saline agglutination test performed in a small test tube. There was no centrifugation, the tests being incubated for a full two hours at room temperature before being interpreted, without shaking, by evaluating the appearance of the pattern formed by the sedimented cell button. In a negative test, the cells settled into a compact, smooth-edged button, while a positive reaction resulted in spreading of the cells over a wider area of the tube bottom, invariably with a crenated edge which, as

John Case, FIMLS, Director of Regulatory Affairs, Gamma Biologicals, Inc., Houston, Texas.

99

incubation proceeded, tended to fold in to give an uneven or angular contour to the edge of the cell button.

The first human example of anti-Rh, described in 1939 by Levine and Stetson,[5] and other early antibodies directed at antigens of the Rh system, were similarly detected and investigated by means of direct agglutination tests performed with simple suspensions of red blood cells in isotonic saline. Weiner and Peters[6] even reported they found the reactions given by some human anti-Rh serums to be improved by incubation in the cold, or by chilling for a few minutes with subsequent centrifugation and gentle shaking before examination for agglutination.

The pioneer investigators soon discovered that results obtained with human anti-Rh sera were not consistently reliable. Variable reactions were often observed when the same serum was used to test different Rh-positive red cells, or when the same Rh-positive cells were tested with different anti-Rh sera. In testing unknown sera for the presence of suspected anti-Rh, microscopic examination was often advocated to avoid interpreting weak reactions as negative. There appeared to be no constant correlation between the severity of hemolytic disease of the newborn (then called erythroblastosis fetalis), and the strength of anti-Rh antibodies detected in the serum of the mother. Indeed, in some cases where the infant of an Rh-negative mother was apparently suffering from severe hemolytic disease, no anti-Rh could be demonstrated in the maternal serum at all.

In 1944, Race[7] and Wiener[8] independently reported that anti-Rh could exist in a form that could not be detected in a saline agglutination test. Yet the presence of nonagglutinating antibodies in such a serum could be demonstrated through their ability to inhibit the reactions of agglutinating antibodies of the same specificity, presumably by competing for the appropriate antigen sites on the red cells. Wiener's "Blocking Test,"[8] though scarcely approaching the level of sensitivity achieved by present-day techniques for the detection of blood group antibodies, is nevertheless of historic interest as sometimes having led to successful diagnosis when the time-honored test method failed. The test was performed by mixing equal volumes of the serum suspected to contain incomplete Rh antibodies and a 2% suspension of known Rh-positive red cells in saline in a test tube and incubating for 30-60 minutes at 38 C. Saline-agglutinating anti-Rh serum, suitably diluted to give a reaction of intermediate strength with the indicator cells, was then added and, after incubation for a further 30-60 minutes, the cells were examined for agglutination. As a control, the same indicator cells were first incubated with a serum known not to contain Rh antibodies,

100

then incubated with the same diluted saline-agglutinating anti-Rh serum. If the cells in the tube containing the test showed no agglutination, or if the degree of agglutination in the test was perceptibly weaker than the agglutination observed in the control test, the test serum was confirmed to have contained nonagglutinating anti-Rh.

"Complete" and "Incomplete" Antibodies

It has long been an accepted belief that antibody-mediated hemagglutination occurs in two stages. When antibodies specific for red cell surface antigens are brought into proximity with red cells possessing the appropriate antigen, individual antibody molecules bind to specific receptor sites on red cells. The second stage, which can be occurring concurrently with the first, involves crosslinking through the attachment of cell-bound antibody to receptors on other cells. The concept of crosslinking, or lattice-formation, was originally proposed in the context of the immune precipitation reaction by Marrack[9] in 1938, and was inherent in the notion invoked in the mid-1940s to explain the failure of some Rh antibodies to produce detectable agglutination of saline-suspended red cells, while evidently being fully capable of blocking their agglutination by antibodies that ordinarily would agglutinate them. Such "blocking" antibodies were considered to be "univalent" (referred to by some authors as "monovalent"), or "incomplete," in the sense that they were viewed as possessing only a single antigen-combining site and were thus able to accomplish only the first stage of agglutination. Since the absence of more than one antigen-combining site on each antibody molecule would prevent the reaction from proceeding to the second stage, agglutination would be unable to take place. At the same time, red cells incubated with a serum containing incomplete antibodies could be expected to become unagglutinable by serums containing "bivalent" or "complete" antibodies of the same specificity, as their receptor sites for that antigen would now be blocked, effectively preventing the subsequent participation of the cells in either the first or second stages of the agglutination reaction with antibodies of that specificity.

The terms "incomplete antibody" and (perhaps to a somewhat lesser extent) "complete antibody" have persisted in common usage to the present day, although the misconception on which they were founded has become evident with clearer understanding of the structure of immunoglobulin molecules. Antibodies capable of agglutinating antigen-positive red cells in a saline test system belong for the most part to the IgM class of immunoglobulin, while those that do not

101

agglutinate are predominantly IgG. The failure of IgG molecules to bring about direct agglutination is attributable to their size in relation to the distance that separates red cells suspended in an electrolyte solution. Crosslinking by IgM antibodies occurs readily because the IgM molecule is large enough to span the distance between individual red cells in the test system. The IgG molecule, on the other hand, though indeed being "complete" in regard to possessing the two antigen-combining sites needed to permit crosslinking between separate red cells, is only able to bind to one red cell at a time when the test medium is saline, as no second cell can come close enough to be reached by the other antigen-combining site. Accordingly, the antigen-antibody reaction is limited to the first stage and, in the absence of crosslinking, agglutination fails to take place.

Methods by which IgG antibodies can be made to agglutinate antigen-positive red cells include the employment of a second antibody to form agglutinates by crosslinking cell-bound IgG; the chemical modification of the IgG molecule to increase its flexibility; and the achievement of a reduction in the intercellular distance, either by treating the red cell surface with an enzyme or by adjusting the composition of the test medium. Substances used to adjust the test medium as a means of promoting hemagglutination are called potentiators. Their number includes a variety of natural and synthetic polymers which have been used for 30 years and more, either separately or in combination, to yield the desired effect by a mechanism it would seem reasonable to suppose is essentially similar for them all.

Potentiation by Human Serum or Plasma

In 1945, Diamond and Abelson[10] introduced a slide test they reported to be more reliable for the detection of "incomplete" Rh antibodies than the then-current saline test system. The test was performed by mixing equal parts of the test serum and anticoagulated Rh-positive whole blood on a microscope slide, then using a 25-watt electric bulb—forerunner of the now-familiar Rh viewbox—to provide both warmth to incubate the test mixture and light to examine for agglutination. It was emphasized that a thick drop of blood was a necessity for reliable results, and it was at first suggested that once-washed cells resuspended in saline to a concentration of 40-50% would serve in place of whole blood. Wiener[11] later reported, and the original authors concurred,[12] that impaired sensitivity was the result if the indicator cells were suspended in saline, and that the maintenance of a total protein test environment was essential for satisfactory sensitivity. If washed cells were to be used at all, it was agreed they must be resuspended in human plasma or serum.

It is a limitation of slide tests for hemagglutination that the reaction mixture has a tendency to dry out, especially at the edges, leading to aggregation of the red cells that could be mistaken for a positive test reaction, especially when, as with many sera containing incomplete Rh antibodies, only relatively feeble agglutination could be observed. As a safeguard, Diamond and Abelson recommended a parallel control test in which the test serum was incubated with a drop of known Rh-negative whole blood, to facilitate comparison in the event of doubt. Drying of the reactants on an open slide understandably depends on the duration of incubation required to permit agglutination to develop; and the necessity for incubation at above room temperature, as in Rh tests, tends to aggravate the risk of false positive interpretation. This consideration provides what is possibly a major reason for the fact that tube tests are generally preferred to slide tests for the detection of most hemagglutination reactions.

The "Conglutination Test" of Wiener[11] simply applied the enhancing effect of human plasma or serum to a tube test procedure. As in the slide test, the cell suspension was made in compatible human plasma, except that instead of the heavy concentration of cells needed for a slide test, a 2% suspension was made. Equal parts of the test serum and the plasma-suspended cells were then incubated together in a tube for one hour, at the end of which time the sedimented cells were examined for agglutination. Wiener hypothesized that the effectiveness of human plasma (which he considered to be superior to serum for the test) was due to the presence of a heat-stable colloidal aggregate of proteins called conglutinin, which had the ability to cause red cells to agglutinate once they had become sensitized with univalent Rh antibody. The word "conglutinin" was originally introduced in 1908 by Bordet and Streng[16] to describe the component of normal bovine serum they considered to be responsible for the ability of bovine serum to agglutinate red cells that had been sensitized with antibody and complement, to which phenomenon Wiener perceived a parallel in the potentiation of Rh agglutination by plasma.

Bovine Albumin and Other Viscous Solutions as Potentiators of Agglutination

Recognition of the fact that bovine albumin would assist "incomplete" Rh antibodies to agglutinate antigen-positive red cells came almost as soon as the discovery that such antibodies existed. Diamond and Denton[13] studied the ability of bovine or human albumin to enable the reactions of "incomplete" Rh antibodies to be seen as agglutination, and developed a tube technique utilizing 20% bovine albumin as the cell-suspending medium in tests for the detection of Rh antibodies. Later, Cameron and Diamond[14] studied the enhancement of Rh agglutination by human and bovine albumin, and proposed that albumin could be employed as a diluent for Rh globulin preparations prepared by fractionation from Rh-immune serums, which were being used at the time for Rh typing procedures.

Continuing to study the phenomenon of conglutination, Wiener et al[15] discovered that bovine albumin could be utilized to "fortify" the conglutinin component of human plasma. By titrating "univalent" Rh antibodies in human plasma, then testing the dilutions with Rh-positive red cells suspended to a 2% concentration in various mixtures of human plasma and albumin, Wiener came to the conclusion that a cell-suspending medium consisting of four parts of human plasma to one part of 25% albumin provided greater sensitivity than 25% albumin used alone, and showed a fourfold increase in the conglutination titer over human plasma used alone.

Early Hypotheses

Several possible explanations were offered for the ability of albumin to promote immune hemagglutination. Race[7] considered that the supposed structural defect of the "incomplete" antibody molecule was in some way corrected in a test system containing a high concentration of protein or some other suitable colloid, while Wiener[17] modified his earlier hypothesis about conglutination with the proposition that protein-enhanced agglutination is brought about by the adsorption of albumin molecules to the red cells, resulting in a reduction in the net surface charge. Such a reduction, Wiener reasoned, enabled "univalent" antibodies to produce agglutination; while "bivalent" antibodies themselves reduced the surface charge, and were able to produce agglutination unaided. In the meantime, other polymers found to be promising as agents that might be used to enhance agglutination included gelatin,[13,18] gum acacia,[19] dextran,[20,21] and polyvinylpyrrolidone (PVP).[22]

The suggestion that the molecular size of immunoglobulin in relation to intercellular distance might be involved in permitting or preventing hemagglutination came first from Hirszfeld and Dubiski,[23] who showed that bringing red cells into closer proximity by centrifugation at high speed could induce agglutination by antibodies that would not ordinarily agglutinate saline-suspended cells. Without offering an explanation of the possible mechanism, these authors proposed that the distance between suspended red cells was reduced by colloid solutions such as bovine albumin, to such a degree that the smaller molecules of "incomplete" antibody could achieve the cross-linking needed to produce agglutination. This concept now goes unquestioned, but there have been conflicting scientific explanations to account for the forces holding red cells apart when suspended in electrolyte solutions, and in turn for the mechanisms whereby these forces are overcome in the various test procedures that have proved effective in promoting hemagglutination by some IgG antibodies.

These matters are of little practical interest at bench level in the routine blood grouping laboratory, where reasonably consistent reliability of effect understandably inhibits the desire to question cause. The effectiveness of potentiators was discovered empirically to begin with, by investigators who ascribed their success to a variety of factors that remained in the realm of speculation. Variables such as optimal concentrations, proportions and choice of molecular weight were determined by trial and error, rather than by separate, systematic applications of well-established or thoroughly-understood scientific principles. Inevitably, thanks to the scientific curiosity of humankind, explanations supported by experimental evidence continued to be sought. Inevitably, thanks to the diversity of human ingenuity, the search led in different directions, and yielded data that lent itself to interpretation in different ways.

The end result—to date, at least—has been the development of at least two schools of thought about the nature of forces chiefly responsible for maintaining the separation of red cells in suspension, and to perhaps three or more about the principles by which polymers overcome these forces to a degree that permits hemagglutination to occur. Although the second stage of the hemagglutination reaction has already been addressed in this seminar, it is scarcely possible to review developments in the use of potentiators without considering, once again, the beliefs that exist concerning their mode or modes of action.

Current Hypotheses

Zeta Potential

In 1965, Pollack et al[24] presented convincing experimental data to support the idea that the distance separating red cells in suspension in an electrolyte solution is dependent on the zeta potential at the "surface of shear," also known as the "slipping plane." Since red cells are

105

negatively charged, their suspension in a salt solution results in the formation around each cell of a cloud of positively charged ions, which gradually diminishes in density towards its outer boundary, this being the slipping plane. As each red cell moves in the suspension, the cation cloud moves with it and repels the similar cloud surrounding adjacent cells, with the effect that the slipping plane of each determines the nearest distance to which any one red cell can approach any other. The zeta potential is the difference in potential between the negatively-charged cell surface and the outer boundary of the kinetically bound cation cloud, and an effect of reducing zeta potential is to bring the suspended red cells into closer proximity.

Zeta potential is inversely proportional to the ionic strength and the dielectric constant of the suspending medium. Thus, since it is possible to calculate zeta potential from the electrophoretic mobility of red cells suspended in a buffer solution of known ionic strength and dielectric constant, the effect on zeta-potential of certain polymers used as additives to the suspending medium can be calculated.

Bovine albumin and three synthetic polymers, polyvinylpyrrolidone, Ficoll® and dextran, were shown to reduce the zeta potential by raising the dielectric constant—at least in the immediate vicinity of the individual red cells, if not of the bulk medium. The effect may be visualized as being caused by dispersal of charged particles resulting from the orientation of the macromolecules within the cation cloud surrounding each red cell, leading to dissipation of the charge and a consequent lessening of the repulsive forces holding the cells apart. No evidence was found to suggest that these substances influence the surface charge of the red cell.

By utilizing appropriate concentrations of the polymer solutions to achieve dielectric increments resulting in selected zeta potentials, and by comparing the agglutinability of the suspended red cells by IgG anti-D, Pollack and his associates determined that the critical zeta potential at which the cells are brought into sufficient proximity to be agglutinated by the IgG antibody is approximately −13.0 millivolts. Further reduction (to about −8 mV) was considered necessary for optimum agglutination, and a tendency was observed for the red cells to aggregate spontaneously if the zeta potential was brought below −7 mV. The reactivity of saline-agglutinating anti-D was also shown to be dependent on zeta potential, with −23 mV being the critical level above which agglutination is unable to occur and −18 mV the level below which no further enhancement of agglutination is demonstrated.

Pollack and his co-workers noted that, while other substances than polymers (notably amino acids, such as epsilon-amino caproic acid) might have the dielectric properties needed to effect a reduction in zeta potential, the concentration required to achieve the desired effect on the intercellular distance would defeat the objective by interfering with the ability of the immunoglobulin molecule to bind to the specific antigen receptors on the cells. Similarly with manipulating ionic strength as a means of reducing zeta potential, as primary binding of antibody to antigen occurs most readily at an ionic strength actually lower than that of isotonic saline. The increase in salt concentration that would be needed to bring the zeta potential into the critical range for agglutination to occur would be such that antigen-antibody interaction would tend to be inhibited altogether.

The elegant study by Pollack et al included measurements of the change in the electrophoretic mobility of red cells achieved by the methods of enzyme treatment commonly used in blood group serology. The results were calculated to represent reductions in zeta potential ranging from 20% for trypsin to 54% for ficin. Since the treatment of red cells with certain enzymes removes the surface sialic acid groups on which the negative charge of the cell is largely dependent, the efficacy of enzymes in making antigen-positive red cells agglutinable by some IgG antibodies could be explained by the resulting reduction in zeta potential, rather than being primarily due to increased exposure of antigen following enzyme treatment as originally suggested by Wiener and Katz,[25] or to an enhancement of the rate of association between antigen and antibody as proposed by Hughes-Jones et al.[26]

Water of Hydration

The proposition that the separation of suspended red cells is influenced by tightly-bound water at the cell surface was advanced in 1964 by Hummel.[27] This concept is favored by Greenwalt and Steane,[28-30] and by Good and Wood[31-33]; and experimental evidence presented by Hughes-Jones et al[34] would be consistent with such an idea. Investigators who are convinced that water of hydration plays a major role in maintaining the distance between red cells in suspension are not entirely unanimous in their beliefs about the precise mechanism, but the explanation presented by Steane[29,35] is that water is bound tightly by the glycoproteins of the red cell membrane, particularly by the sialic acid terminal residues, and that this water forms an integral part of the membrane. The natural propensity of suspended red cells to aggregate is opposed by a combination of the negative electrical charge associated with the terminal sialic acid groups, and steric hindrance resulting from the bound water.

Removal of sialic acid (as may be achieved by treatment with enzymes) reduces both the surface charge and the amount of water at the cell surface, while the presence of macromolecules in the suspension causes disruption and dispersal of bound water. In either case, there may be multiple effects contributing to the enhancement of agglutination. Since the antigen-antibody reaction is impeded by competition with the cell surface for the bound water of the membrane, the release of water provides the entropy component to lend impetus to antigen-antibody interaction, which is further aided by the concurrent removal of steric hindrance and, under optimal conditions, agglutination is able to take place.

Some Alternative Suggestions

An apparent contradiction of the premise that IgG molecules cannot span the distance that separates individual cells is the fact that some IgG antibodies readily agglutinate antigen-positive red cells suspended in saline. IgG antibodies of anti-A and anti-B specificity, in particular, possess the ability to produce direct agglutination of saline-suspended red cells positive for the particular antigen, as do some examples of IgG anti-D when tested in a saline medium with cells of the -D- phenotype. An acceptable explanation for these exceptions might be that they are made possible by the greater number of the relevant antigen sites on the cells concerned, having regard to the fact that the mere attachment of antibody to antigen on the cell results in some reduction of the net negative surface charge. As early as 1926, Schroeder[36] reported a fall in zeta potential when group A and group B cells were sensitized with anti-A and anti-B, respectively; and Pollack et al[24] in their study confirmed that antibody sensitization, whether by IgM or by IgG antibodies, reduces the net surface charge, which in turn results in a corresponding reduction in zeta potential. The antigen-antibody reaction is similarly considered to cause a release of cell-bound water. Given that the extent of either of these effects is likely to be proportional to the number of antigen sites to which antibody is bound, this may be sufficient in these cases for the cells to be agglutinated, whichever phenomenon is considered to be responsible; while in antigen-antibody interactions involving fewer receptors the critical level may not be reached for agglutination to occur.

Reasoning based on heavy antigen density cannot be invoked to account for the fact that some IgG examples of anti-K produce direct agglutination of saline-suspended K-positive cells. The number of K sites on the red cell has been reported by Hughes-Jones et al[37,38] to be substantially fewer than the number of D sites, yet Stratton[39 (p33)] reported successful K-typing by a layering technique involving only a saline suspension of red cells and no potentiator, and Grove-Rasmussen et al[40] found cells suspended in whole serum to be suitable for detecting eight examples of anti-K by direct agglutination, although suspension of the cells in 20% bovine albumin would not result in agglutination.

The parts played by zeta potential and water of hydration as the only factors contributing to maintaining the separation of red cells in suspension have each been questioned, mainly on the grounds that there are inconsistencies left unexplained by one hypothesis or the other, or in some cases by both. For example, Stratton et al[41] determined that an IgG anti-D serum showed a very much higher titration endpoint against D-positive red cells treated with cysteine-activated papain than against the same cells treated with neuraminidase. Even though neuraminidase and papain had been used to achieve about the same reduction in net negative surface charge in the experiment, the effects of the two enzymes on the agglutinability of the cells by IgG anti-D proved to be very different. Indeed, even when the neuraminidase treatment was extended to achieve a greater reduction in surface charge than was achieved with papain, the same IgG anti-D serum still showed a much lower titer with the neuraminidase-treated cells than with papain-treated cells. The conclusion was reached that a reduction of zeta potential is not the factor of greatest importance when enzyme treatment causes red cells to become agglutinable by IgG antibodies of appropriate specificity. It was suggested that, since neuraminidase selectively removes N-acetyl neuraminic acid from the cell surface, whereas proteases also remove the polypeptide stem, the greater effect on agglutinability by papain and other proteases has to do with the removal of steric hindrance. No comment was made by Stratton et al on the mechanism by which polymers promote agglutination but, since the zeta potential hypothesis offers to explain this and the effect of enzymes on the same basis, their conclusion introduced an element of doubt that a reduction in zeta potential was the explanation for either.

Another comparison between papain-treated and neuraminidase-treated cells was made by Voak et al,[42] who extended their investigation to include both saline and bovine albumin test procedures, and an ultrastructural study of D-positive red cells incubated with ferritin-labeled anti-D. Examination of the albumin and papain tests by electron microscopy showed powerful agglutination of the red cells with large areas of cell-to-cell contact involving 90% or more of the total cell surface area, whereas the neuraminidase test showed only loose, weak agglutinates with relatively smaller areas of contact involving 50% or less of the surface area. These findings appeared to indicate that the net force of aggregation is considerably weaker between neuraminidase-treated cells than between either untreated cells in the albumin test or between papain-treated cells, even though neuraminidase achieves the same reduction in zeta potential as papain. This would be confirmation of the conclusion that a reduction in zeta potential is not a prominent factor in the enhancement of Rh agglutination by enzymes, and would apply the same doubt to the rule of albumin.

The purpose of attaching a ferritin label to the anti-D used in this study was to determine the distribution of D antigen sites on the cells in the different test systems. When the serum-cell mixtures were examined by electron microscopy, clustering of the ferritin was seen on the enzyme-treated cells (both papain and neuraminidase), which suggested that enzymes make agglutination possible by producing localized clusters of antigen sites, and that the greater efficacy of papain (and perhaps other proteases) in making red cells agglutinable may be due to the lessening of steric hindrance resulting from the removal of the polypeptide stem.

No antigen clustering was observed in the albumin test, nor on the surfaces of the sensitized but unagglutinated cells in the saline test. In both cases, the ferritin was observed to be distributed evenly over the cell surface, indicating the points at which the labeled anti-D had attached. From this evidence, Vodak and his associates concluded that albumin must act to potentiate agglutination by a different mechanism than enzymes and that, judging from the appearance of the agglutinates, this might be by increasing the areas of cell-to-cell contact, thereby improving the likelihood of multiple bridging between cells, which was reported by Greenbury et al[43] to be an important element of the hemagglutination reaction, at least by rabbit IgG. It was believed that this effect is no more caused by the dispersal of cell-bound water than by a reduction of zeta potential, as an earlier study by Voak and Downie[44] had furnished evidence suggesting that disturbance of water of hydration is not a factor contributing to hemagglutination. It was suggested that albumin may cause weak transient aggregation of the suspended cells which, if already sensitized by antibody, become agglutinated because the brief contact with adjacent cells enables the cell-bound IgG to form multiple crosslinks if the site density of the antigen in question is sufficient.

The zeta potential theory as it applies to the effectiveness of polymers in causing agglutination has also been challenged by Brooks and Seaman,[45] whose experimental studies led to the conclusion that, far from decreasing zeta potential, dextran actually increases it, sometimes to a considerable degree that is dependent on the molecular weight and concentration of dextran present. Findings by Jan and Chien[46] and by Jones[47] support this belief.

Brooks[48] studied the spontaneous cellular aggregation that takes place when washed human red cells are suspended in dextran solutions made in saline, and noted that the phenomenon rises to a peak as the concentration of dextran is increased, then diminishes with further increase in the dextran concentration, followed by disaggregation at even higher concentrations of dextran. The critical concentrations of dextran at which aggregation and disaggregation took place were dependent on the molecular weight of the dextran used. Below 41,000, no aggregation occurred at all; but the higher the molecular weight the lower the concentration of dextran needed to cause aggregation to begin, the greater the intensity of aggregation attained before disaggregation began, and the higher the concentration of dextran required before disaggregation was complete.

Brooks considered that aggregation by dextran is caused by polymer bridging resulting from the adsorption to two cells of dextran molecules large enough to span the intercellular distance, and that disaggregation occurs when the resultant increase in zeta potential reaches a point where the repulsive forces exceed the tendency to aggregate. This phenomenon was hypothesized to be a factor in the enhancement of agglutination by the introduction of dextran into the test system, presumably at a concentration determined to be below that at which nonspecific aggregation would confuse the specificity of the hemagglutination reaction, but sufficient to assist immunoglobulin molecules to form crosslinks between cells. The same explanation would serve for the role of albumin and other polymers in potentiating agglutination, with molecular weight being perhaps the factor of greatest significance in determining the relative efficacy of different polymers in this context. Pollack et al[24] noted that, of the substances they studied, albumin was the least effective in enabling agglutination to occur. It was also the least in terms of molecular asymmetry and weight. The report by Jones et al[49] that polymeric albumin is more effective as a potentiator than the monomer may be a further indication that larger molecules fulfill the function better than smaller ones.

In a review of the subject by van Oss et al,[50,51] it was conceded that zeta potential may play a major role in maintaining the separation of red cells in suspension, but the reduction of zeta potential was considered a factor of minor significance in the potentiation of hemagglutination. Referring to an earlier study[52] on the ability of phagocytes to overcome repulsive forces by means of protrusions from their surfaces, the effect of changes in the morphology of the red cell membrane was thought to be important in aiding agglutination to take place. It was noted that Salsbury and Clark[53] had reported that anti-A causes strong spiculation of group A, D-positive red cells, whereas anti-D does not. This finding had been confirmed by van Oss and Mohn,[54] who noted that this phenomenon appears to occur equally with both IgM and IgG antibodies. If spiculation leads to diminished intercellular distance this, rather than a reduction in zeta potential or water of hydration, could be the main reason why ABO antibodies of the IgG class will readily agglutinate antigen-positive red cells suspended in saline, whereas anti-D, which does not cause spiculation, will not. Van Oss and his co-workers reported their own observation that a 10% solution of dextran (MW 40,000) causes spiculation of red cells that is distinctly visible with the aid of a light microscope, and they suggested that this could be a factor in bringing cells into sufficient proximity for direct hemagglutination by IgG antibodies. Of the variety of factors viewed by these authors as producing the combined effect of enhanced agglutination, those considered of greatest importance were polymer bridging (in itself possibly a cause of the spiculation noted with dextran), and increased colloid-osmotic pressure causing several effects, including changes both in hydration and in the shape of the red cell envelope leading to closer contact between larger surface areas of the cells.

By whatever mode or modes of action polymers enable IgG antibodies to cause direct agglutination of antigen-positive red cells, their practical applications have been most consistently successful in improving the reactions of Rh antibodies. A good number of the "new" blood group antibodies reported since 1945 have proved to be no more capable of agglutinating red cells in an albumin test system than in a saline one. In many cases, the recognition of these antibodies was made possible only by the use of the indirect antiglobulin test,[55] wherein agglutination is brought about by crosslinking of cell-bound immunoglobulin molecules through the use of an animal serum specific for human globulin, rather than through a reduction in intercellular distance.

Although somewhat more susceptible than most direct agglutination test systems to an impairment of sensitivity by imperfections in performance, the antiglobulin technique undoubtedly provides the most reliable means of detecting most IgG antibodies, and for those of Rh specificity is exceeded in sensitivity only by methods involving enzyme premodification of the indicator red cells.

Developments in the Practical Use of Potentiators

From the realization that bovine albumin would potentiate aggluti-nation by so-called incomplete antibodies, practical applications of the principle followed different courses. Most prominent among consider-ations that determined the choice of technique were convenience of use and suitability to serve different purposes. Understandably, hemagglutination tests designed for antigen typing procedures had requirements that differed from those designed for antibody detec-tion. No less understandably, the use of potentiators in antibody detection tests was influenced by the knowledge that their demon-strated effectiveness in producing agglutination by Rh antibodies may not apply to immune antibodies of other specificities.

Potentiation of Antisera for Antigen Typing

The predominant requirement for an antiserum intended as a blood grouping reagent is that the test procedure should yield specific posi-tive and negative reactions with minimal prior preparation of the test sample. This is particularly true in the case of typing for the A, B and D antigens on potential blood transfusion recipients, as the ABO and D antigen status must be determined before appropriate donor blood can be chosen. ABO blood grouping sera present no difficulty in this regard, as anti-A and anti-B are readily available in the form of power-ful direct agglutinins. Antibodies directed at the D antigen, on the other hand, are most abundantly available in the form that, however potent, does not yield direct agglutination of D-positive red cells sus-pended in saline. This means that potentiators must be employed when typing with most anti-D sera, ideally in such a concentration that strong macroscopic agglutination is seen consistently with D-positive red cells, yet that the resulting viscosity does not cause equiv-ocal reactions with D-negative cells.

The earliest applications of bovine albumin as a potentiator of agglu-tination were not entirely suitable for D antigen typing, as the require-ments of reliable specificity and convenience were not met. The slide test method using an anticoagulated whole blood specimen required particular care in choosing the antiserum; while the tube test with a suspension of the test cells that had to be made in bovine albumin was inconvenient and time-consuming. Selected sera containing anti-D could be prediluted in albumin and used to test for the D antigen by the slide or tube test, but a suspension of the test cells in serum remained a necessity, as suspension of the cells in saline had the effect of reducing the strength of agglutination. The tube test also required a period of incubation before being interpreted, which introduced an unwanted delay in obtaining the test result.

Polymers such as gum acacia, dextran and polyvinylpyrrolidone were found to potentiate agglutination at lower concentrations than bovine albumin, but also to have a tendency to cause red cells to aggregate nonspecifically. Combined with bovine albumin in balanced proportions, however, these substances had the effect of reducing the concentration of albumin needed for agglutination to occur, and also of accelerating the reaction. By diluting potent anti-D sera in such a mixture, anti-D blood grouping reagents were prepared that could be used, either with a heavy drop of whole blood on a warm slide, or in a tube with a saline suspension of cells, and would yield strong, rapid and specific reactions comparable with those produced by ABO reagents, with almost the same degree of reliability. The reservation about reliability is due to the fact that any test system that potentiates direct agglutination by IgG antibodies also tends to cause spontaneous agglutination of red cells that have become coated with immunoglobulin in vivo. This is especially true when the test mixture contains a macromolecular additive to accelerate the specific reaction, as this also accelerates the potentially false positive reactions that may occur in patients suffering from some disease states, or who are receiving certain forms of medication, that are associated with sensitization of the red cells by immunoglobulin. Rh antisera prepared in this way, using a variety of different macromolecular additives, have been commercially available for many years. Such sera were used initially with no control test to recognize false reactions due to immunoglobulin coated to the test cells. Later, a somewhat less than adequate parallel control test using bovine albumin was recommended on all specimens tested; more recently, it came to be realized that confident recognition of false positive reactions caused by spontaneous agglutination required that the parallel control test should be carried out with an inert reagent containing bovine albumin and the same macromolecular additive present in the antiserum being controlled, in similar proportions and at comparable concentrations.

In Britain and in other places where commercial antisera were slow to gain acceptance, Rh antigen typings continued to be performed with selected patient sera containing appropriate antibodies. Macromolecular additives did not become widely used and, even in relatively recent times, Rh typing in Britain has been performed largely with selected patient sera absorbed to remove unwanted ABO antibodies, then distributed through the Regional Blood Transfusion Centers to be used either by an enzyme test procedure, by some variation of the Diamond and Denton albumin test, or by a method determined at the particular user's discretion. Tests were (and still are) commonly performed in precipitin tubes (approximately 50 × 6 mm), and the incubation period was commonly up to two hours, as sedimentation by gravity was more favored than centrifugation as a means of bringing the red cells together to maximize completion of the second stage of the agglutination reaction. Testing for D in urgent cases was usually performed by an enzyme method, or else using reagents prepared from serums containing strong direct saline anti-D agglutinins kept in reserve for the purpose, while donor samples and those of patients in nonurgent cases were normally subjected to the more prolonged procedure.

Stratton's Sandwich Technique

In 1956, Stratton[56] introduced a variation of the warm slide test that was quicker and easier to perform than then-current tube testing methods for D-typing, and was less prone to false interpretation due to drying of the reactants than the original open slide procedure. One drop of a suitable serum containing incomplete anti-D was placed on a microscope slide, together with one drop of 30% bovine albumin and one drop of once-washed packed cells from the blood sample to be tested. After mixing the reactants, a second slide was placed on top to form a "sandwich." Any excess fluid exuding from between the two slides was then wiped away and the "sandwich" was incubated at 37 C for 10 minutes before being examined microscopically for agglutination. The sandwich technique, by permitting longer incubation without drying than is possible on an open slide, gave extra sensitivity to the relatively rapid detection of the D antigen with sera that contained IgG anti-D, and required somewhat less potent antibodies than the original slide method. The test was messy to perform, however, and failed to achieve universal adoption (even though the need for precautions against the transmission of hepatitis by human blood products had still to be realized in 1956).

Albumin Replacement

To overcome difficulties caused by viscosity when bovine albumin was used as the medium for suspending the red cells, Dunsford and Bowley[57] introduced the albumin replacement technique in 1955. The test is set up initially as for a saline agglutination test in a 50 × 6 mm

115

tube, using equal volumes of serum and a suspension of red cells in saline. The mixture is incubated at 37 C for 90 minutes, during which time the cells settle into a compact button in the bottom of the tube. At the end of the incubation period, the supernatant serum/saline mixture is very gently removed without disturbing the cell button, and is replaced by a drop of 20% bovine albumin. The test is then reincubated at 37 C for 30 minutes, without mixing to resuspend the cells. It is very important not to disturb the cell button, as the test was designed to be read without centrifugation, and resuspension of the cells at this point would mean they would not settle adequately during the second period of incubation. If the cells become coated with antibody during the first period of incubation (for example if the antiserum is anti-D and the cells are D-positive), they agglutinate spontaneously during the second period of incubation. Agglutination is rapid and powerful because the coated cells are already formed into a compact button before the potentiator is applied, and the effect of bovine albumin percolating between them is to cause strong and abundant crosslinking. The test is usually read by tapping the tube sharply with the finger to dislodge the sedimented cells, which in a test with anti-D come away from the base of the tube in one large, solid clump if they are D-positive, and resuspend easily and evenly if D-negative.

Albumin Layering

The albumin replacement procedure is a highly sensitive technique for the detection of agglutination by incomplete Rh antibodies, but the actual replacement step must be performed with a steady hand or sensitivity is seriously impaired by any disturbance of the cell button at this point. A variation of the original method was introduced in 1959,[58] wherein the supernatant serum/saline is not removed after the first period of incubation, but is merely displaced upwards by allowing a drop of 30% bovine albumin to run down the inside wall of the tube. Because the albumin is considerably more viscous than the original supernate, it flows beneath it and forms a layer immediately over and in contact with the red cell button, thereby achieving the same end as in the original technique, without incurring the risk of prematurely disturbing the sedimented cell button. The choice of 30% bovine albumin instead of the 20% recommended for the original method was made in the mistaken belief that some mixing with the supernate might have a dilution effect that would diminish the sensitivity of the procedure. In practice, however, perfectly satisfactory results may be obtained by adding 20% bovine albumin, as in the albumin replacement method.

Potentiators in Antibody Detection

The earliest bovine albumin test procedures for antibody detection utilized equal parts of the test serum and a suspension of indicator cells in 20% bovine albumin, which were incubated together for up to two hours and then read without centrifugation. Wiener and Hurst[59] and Wiener, Hurst and Sonn-Gordon[15] found a mixture of bovine albumin and human plasma to be more effective than 20% bovine albumin alone, while Stratton and Dimond[60] favored a cell suspending medium comprising equal parts of 30% bovine albumin and whole human serum. In 1958, while conceding that cells suspended in a mixture of serum and albumin were not agglutinated by some IgG antibodies (notably anti-Fy^a, anti-Jk^a and some examples of anti-S), Stratton and Renton[36 (pp37-39)] claimed superiority of the serum and albumin mixture for the detection of Rh antibodies on the ground that prozoning occurred less markedly with potent examples of anti-D than when the cells were suspended in bovine albumin alone, and noted also that anti-K sometimes agglutinated cells suspended in the mixture when no agglutination could be demonstrated with albumin-suspended cells. No explanation was offered for these observations, nor has a convincing one been proposed since; but in any event the use of a serum and albumin mixture to suspend the red cells appears to have been something of a passing fancy. This may be attributable in part to the onus of selecting a suitable source of serologically inert human serum with which to make the mixture, when the albumin replacement technique offered at least equal sensitivity without the inconvenience.

At this time in history, the widespread adoption of the antiglobulin test had already brought the realization that some IgG antibodies do not readily react as direct agglutinins, even in a potentiated test system. To some extent, this realization had made redundant the routine use of potentiators—or, at the very least had relegated bovine albumin to a supernumerary role in the detection of blood group antibodies. While it is true that antibody screening and crossmatching tests continued to include a bovine albumin phase, it was seldom indeed that an antibody was detected by direct agglutination that was not at least as readily recognized in the antiglobulin phase of the test, assuming that the antiglobulin test was performed correctly. The fallibility of the antiglobulin test (especially before the advent of the control using IgG-sensitized cells to verify negative test results) may have been foremost among the reasons why the albumin test was not discontinued altogether, and may have been at least partly responsible for some early reports of Rh antibodies (notably those of anti-E and

117

anti-c specificity) that were said to have shown agglutination in albumin tests, yet to have been undetectable by the indirect antiglobulin test.

The bovine albumin method that came to be most widely used in Britain for antibody detection was the albumin replacement technique or its layering modification. In either case, the test was set up in a 50 × 6 mm tube, and was interpreted microscopically if apparently negative on macroscopic examination after the full two hours incubation. A second 50 × 6 mm tube was used for a parallel saline test to be incubated for two hours at room temperature, and the antiglobulin test was set up in a third, rather larger tube (usually 50 × 12 mm), to facilitate centrifugation during the washing stages to remove unbound globulin. It was common for the test mixture to comprise three or four drops of the test serum to one drop of a 50% suspension of washed indicator cells, and incubation was for two hours at 37 C. No albumin was added, and the heavy concentration of cells was necessitated by the method most frequently used for reading the final reaction after the incubation and washing phases, which was to mix an aliquot of the washed cells with the antiglobulin serum on an opalescent glass tile, then to rock the tile slowly and gently with a circular motion for up to five minutes, while examining continuously over a light source for agglutination.

It is extremely doubtful that IgG antibodies of sufficient potency to be of immediate clinical significance require a full two hours of incubation to achieve adequate sensitization of antigen-positive red cells. Assuming that the first stage of the antigen-antibody reaction would be at least 90% complete within the first 30 minutes of incubation, the remaining 90 minutes of the incubation period would contribute little to the sensitivity of the test, other than to allow sedimentation of the sensitized cells into sufficient proximity for maximal crosslinking to occur. Since centrifugation can be applied to accomplish the same effect within a matter of seconds, the test procedure can be shortened considerably without a loss of sensitivity.

This philosophy had a considerable influence on the evolution of serological testing in the United States, where it was found convenient to utilize centrifugation as a means of developing the second stage of the agglutination reaction and thereby to shorten the duration of incubation in tests for the detection of blood group antibodies. The application of the same principle to the development of agglutination by the antiglobulin reagent meant that the heavier cell suspension needed for a slide test did not have to be considered, and it was accordingly possible to combine the albumin and antiglobulin test procedures. By proceeding to wash the cells in the albumin test after incubation, centrifugation and examination for direct agglutination, then adding the antiglobulin, centrifuging and examining again for agglutination, the two test procedures could be carried out simultaneously in one test tube.

The quest for simplicity and convenience in the performance of antibody detection tests led in turn to a development that has unfortunately compromised the effectiveness of bovine albumin as a potentiator of direct agglutination. The test procedure in which the test serum, a saline suspension of red cells and bovine albumin are incubated together is substantially less sensitive than the albumin replacement or albumin layering methods for detecting direct agglutination by Rh antibodies of the IgG class. Although the presence of bovine albumin has been noted by Stroup and MacIlroy[61] to enhance the sensitivity of the antiglobulin test itself, the concentration of protein achieved by mixing two drops of even 30% bovine albumin with two drops of serum and one drop of saline-suspended cells is only approximately 14.5%, which appears to be below the optimum required for the potentiation of direct agglutination. When 22% bovine albumin is used for the test procedure the protein concentration in the test mixture barely exceeds 11%, so it may not be surprising that Rh antibodies are commonly found to have substantially lower titration values as direct agglutinins in the albumin test than at the antiglobulin phase. It should be noted here that, based on studies by the early investigators, the total protein concentration may not be the critical factor. It was believed, however, that the introduction of an aqueous fluid into the test system had an adverse effect on the sensitivity of the test. It does appear, at any rate, that addition of a cell suspension in saline (or in the suspending medium used in commercial reagent red blood cells) tends to interfere with the ability of IgG Rh antibodies to produce agglutination in the albumin test. When bovine albumin is used by the albumin replacement or layering methods, the titer of Rh antibodies is invariably higher than in the albumin test using a saline suspension of cells, and is most often the same as that observed in the antiglobulin test. This is illustrated in Table 1, which shows the results obtained when dilutions of a serum containing anti-D are prepared in AB serum and then tested against D-positive cells using different test procedures.

Some enhancement of direct agglutination by incomplete Rh antibodies can be achieved by using a "washed button" of the indicator cells in the test procedure instead of a suspension in saline (or reagent red blood cells directly from the vial). One drop of the cell suspension

119

Table 1.—Comparison of Reactions Obtained When Dilutions of an anti-D Serum (She.) made in Group AB Serum Were Tested by a Variety of Test Procedures Against Red Cells of the Phenotype CcDee.

Test Mixture	Reciprocal of Dilutions of Anti-D Serum (in Group AB Serum)									
	2	4	8	16	32	64	128	256	512	1024
2 drops of diluted serum + 1 drop of 3% cell suspension in saline. No additives. Incubation for 15 minutes at 37 C, spun and read.	(+)	0	0	0	0	0	0	0	0	0
Same test, converted to antiglobulin phase and read.	4+	4+	4+	3+	3+	3+	2+	1+	0	0
2 drops of diluted serum + 1 drop of 3% cell suspension in saline + 2 drops of 22% bovine albumin solution. Incubation for 15 minutes at 37 C, spun and read.	3+	2+	1+	(+)	0	0	0	0	0	0
Same test, converted to antiglobulin phase and read.	4+	4+	4+	3+	3+	2+	2+	1+	(+)	0
2 drops of diluted serum + 1 drop of 3% cell suspension in saline + 2 drops of 30% bovine albumin solution. Incubation for 15 minutes at 37 C, spun and read.	4+	3+	1+	(+)	0	0	0	0	0	0
Same test, converted to antiglobulin phase and read.	4+	4+	4+	4+	3+	3+	2+	1+	(+)	0
1 drop of diluted serum + drop of 3% cell suspension in 30% bovine albumin solution. Incubation for 30 minutes at 37 C, spun and read.	4+	4+	3+	2+	1+	(+)	w	0	0	0
Albumin Layering Method 1 drop of diluted serum + 1 drop of 3% cell suspension in saline. Incubation for 60 minutes at 37 C. One drop of 20% bovine albumin added (gently down side of tube to layer over cell button). Incubated further 5 minutes at 37 C. No mix. Read after tapping. No spin.	4+	4+	4+	3+	3+	2+	2+	1+	0	0

is placed in a tube, which is then filled with saline and centrifuged. The saline is removed as completely as possible, and the dry cell button is resuspended in two drops of bovine albumin solution. The purpose of the washing step is not so much to wash the cells as to facilitate the replacement of the original suspending medium by albumin with minimal dilution.

The albumin layering method, though not recommended as consistently reliable for the detection of IgG antibodies outside the Rh system, is occasionally able to detect examples of anti-Fy[a] and anti-K as direct agglutinins, which is seldom possible in a test system where the indicator cells are suspended in bovine albumin before being added to the serum. The advantage possessed by the layering method in this regard, and indeed an explanation for its greater sensitivity in detecting agglutination by Rh antibodies, may be that the sensitized cells are already sedimented before the potentiating effect of bovine

120

albumin is applied, which may simplify the formation of strong cross-linking by promoting larger areas of cell-to-cell contact, even when the density of the relevant antigen sites is less than that of the Rh antigens. The albumin layering method can easily be performed without incubating for a total period of two hours. Adequate sensitization and sedimentation of the red cells occurs with most antibodies in one hour or less, and in practice the second phase of incubation (after adding albumin) can be shortened to five minutes without significantly affecting the strength of agglutination. Indeed, the test can be performed in a 75 × 10 mm test tube to facilitate further shortening of incubation by centrifugation after 30 minutes incubation, whereafter albumin can be allowed to layer over the cell button and the test read after a further five minutes at 37 C. The usual serological centrifuge is unsuitable for this adaptation of the test, as the head holds the tubes in such a manner that the cell button is deposited at an angle to the base of the tube, which creates difficulty in layering albumin evenly over the cells. A centrifuge of the "swing-out" type deposits the red cells into a compact button in the base of the tube, just as occurs by gravity during incubation, and the subsequent layering of albumin can be achieved in the same manner as in the original test.

Macromolecular Additives in the Detection of Unexpected Antibodies

The addition of macromolecular additives to bovine albumin as a means of accelerating direct agglutination by IgG antibodies appears to have been largely confined in its application to the preparation of reagent antiserums. Except in relatively recent times, when the same principle has been applied on a somewhat limited scale in the formulation of several commercial low ionic strength additive solutions, bovine albumin has been the only potentiator widely used in detection tests for unexpected antibodies. In their zeta potential study, Pollack et al[24] found that strong direct agglutination by several examples of anti-Fy[a] and anti-K could be demonstrated using Ficoll®, dextran and polyvinylpyrrolidone, but only at concentrations that caused some degree of nonspecific aggregation of the cells. The proneness of synthetic polymers to cause spontaneous aggregation of red cells undoubtedly had some influence on the common consent by which bovine albumin continued to be the preferred potentiating medium for antibody detection tests performed manually, as the situation is not precisely the same as that in which the formulation of the high-protein diluent is deliberately chosen to be optimal for a particular antiserum. In a reagent to be used in tests with an infinite number and variety of

121

unknown sera, it would be difficult to achieve optimal potentiation of agglutination and yet avoid an unacceptable level of nonspecificity.

Perhaps of greatest promise towards an improvement in the sensitivity of direct agglutination tests for the detection of IgG antibodies was the discovery[49] that polymers of bovine albumin itself enhance agglutination. By substituting polymerized bovine albumin at a protein concentration of around 24% for the 22% bovine albumin most frequently used as an additive to routine antibody detection tests, the ability of the test system to detect Rh antibodies by direct agglutination prior to the antiglobulin phase is dramatically improved. Providing the proportions of polymer to monomer are kept within bounds (up to a maximum of 15% polymer has been suggested), spontaneous aggregation does not cause difficulty due to nonspecificity, and the larger polymerized molecules presumably act in a similar manner to the synthetic polymers used in reagent antisera to overcome the disadvantage created by using red cells suspended in an aqueous fluid for the test.

Macromolecules in Automated Antibody Detection

Although synthetic polymers have not been extensively used in manual tests for the detection of blood group antibodies, hemagglutination tests performed on the Technicon AutoAnalyzer® have for some years employed macromolecular additives to promote agglutination by both IgM and IgG antibodies. Ficoll®, methyl cellulose, dextran, polyvinylpyrrolidone and other polymers have all been applied successfully in the automated procedure to produce strong agglutination, even by antibodies (such as anti-Fy^a) that in manual tests can be made to yield direct agglutination only with difficulty, and are ordinarily only capable of being detected reliably by the indirect antiglobulin test.

The ability of positively charged macromolecules such as Polybrene® and protamine to cause spontaneous aggregation of human red cells was applied by Rosenfield et al[62] and by Lalezari[63,64] to automated hemagglutination tests in the AutoAnalyzer. The effect was the achievement of greatly-enhanced detectability of IgG antibodies, which for those in the Rh and Duffy systems was reported to exceed the sensitivity of the indirect antiglobulin test by one hundredfold; yet, for a reason unexplained, to be only equal in sensitivity to the antiglobulin test for antibodies of the Kell system. The test involves incubation of serum and cells in an acidified low ionic strength medium, followed by aggregation with Polybrene or protamine, which serves the same purpose as centrifugation in manual test procedures, as it brings the cells together to facilitate strong crosslinking by cell-bound immunoglobulin. The manner in which Polybrene and protamine overcome the normal forces of repulsion between suspended red cells may not be the same as that by which other polymers exert this effect. It is tempting to believe, since these molecules carry a positive electrical charge, that aggregation is caused by neutralization of the net negative surface charge of the red cells, but Greenwalt and Steane[25] demonstrated that even negatively charged molecules, such as those of N-acetyl neuraminic acid itself, cause some spontaneous aggregation of red cells. Charge neutralization may play a part—albeit possibly a minor one—accompanied by changes in hydration resulting in complex coacervation between red cells and the polycation molecules, as explained by van Oss et al.[51,52] By whatever mechanism polycations induce spontaneous aggregation, the effect is almost instantly reversible upon the addition of a hypertonic salt solution, whereupon the normal repulsive forces between cells is restored and aggregation disperses. If the cells have become sensitized with antibody during prior incubation in the automated test system, the period of close cell-to-cell contact during aggregation enables crosslinking to occur, and the red cells remain agglutinated instead of dispersing when hypertonic sodium citrate is introduced into the system.

Application of Polycation Aggregation in Manual Antibody Tests

Protamine appears to have been tried in Germany[65,66] during the 1950s to aid in potentiation of direct agglutination by Rh antibodies in manual tests, but if the practice has persisted it has not spread. It seems likely that predictable difficulty in interpreting negative tests would have offset any benefit in terms of improved sensitivity. More recently, an adaptation of the automated antibody detection test using low ionic strength incubation and protamine aggregation has been proposed for use in a manual procedure by Rosenfield et al.[67] The low ionic polycation (LIP) test for augmentation of hemagglutination promises increased sensitivity for the detection of IgG antibodies as direct agglutinins, but is somewhat more cumbersome than conventional manual techniques and may lack popular appeal for that reason.

The LIP test is performed in a series of separate phases, commencing with incubation at low ionic strength for five minutes at 37 C. The tube is then centrifuged and the supernate is replaced with a solution of protamine sulfate in glycine, which causes massive aggregation. After brief incubation, the protamine is removed and disaggregation is brought about by adding a phosphate buffer/saline solution. Red cells which have adsorbed antibody during the incubation phase remain agglutinated, but if no antigen-antibody reaction took place during incubation the red cells resuspend more or less evenly. A negative control test utilizing (preferably) an inert group AB serum is recommended to facilitate comparison of reactions obtained with unknown serums, and a hand lens is preferable to a microscope for the examination to determine whether the test is positive or negative, as small aggregates commonly persist in negative tests. Examination for direct agglutination may be followed by washing the cells (two changes of saline are sufficient, as the supernate has already been removed twice) the addition of antiglobulin serum, centrifugation and reexamination for agglutination, as in the conventional antiglobulin test.

It will be apparent that the LIP augmentation test involves more manipulation than existing antibody detection procedures, and that a key factor in being able to interpret test results reliably may be the achievement of uniformity in the agitation applied at the disaggregation phase. This may be accomplished best by some mechanical means, but confident mastery of the test procedure would appear to call for special skill.

Enhancement of the Indirect Antiglobulin Reaction

Up to this point, attention has been paid solely to potentiatiors of direct agglutination, which achieve their effect by reducing intercellular distance, thereby promoting the second stage of the hemagglutination reaction. The sensitivity of the indirect antiglobulin test is not influenced by intercellular distance, but by the extent and rate of association between antibody and antigen during the first stage of the reaction. With the exception of the report by Stroup and McIlroy[61] on the ability of bovine albumin to enhance the sensitivity of the indirect antiglobulin test, substances used to potentiate direct agglutination have shown little measurable effect in this regard. In retrospect, the observations of Stroup and McIlroy may have been attributable to a reduction in the ionic strength of the test system when bovine albumin was added, rather than to an effect brought about by albumin as such.

A reduced ionic strength environment during incubation was shown by several investigators[66-71] to achieve a markedly increased rate of antigen-antibody association, but the first practical application of the principle in routine antibody detection was reported in 1974 by

Löw and Messeter.[72] In place of physiologic saline as the suspending medium for the indicator cells, the use of a low ionic strength solution (LISS) containing glycine and 0.03M sodium chloride was found to increase the rate of antigen-antibody binding to such a degree that incubation could be reduced to a mere five minutes at 37C without a loss of sensitivity in detecting blood group antibodies by the indirect antiglobulin test. This observation has since been confirmed by a number of other investigators,[73-79] and the technique—or some modification of it—has become the routine procedure for antibody detection in many laboratories.

In a test system using LISS-suspended red cells there is no potentiation of direct agglutination, so the reliable detection of IgG antibodies depends wholly on the correct performance of the indirect antiglobulin test. A few commercially available low ionic strength reagents are designed as additives to facilitate the conversion of a conventional test system into a low ionic one without the inconvenience of having to make a special suspension of red cells. Other low ionic strength additive solutions include a variety of macromolecules into the formulation, with the object of potentiating direct agglutination by some IgG antibodies, as well as enhancing the indirect antiglobulin test by creating a low ionic environment during the incubation phase of the test.

It does seem that incubation at low ionic strength improves antibody detection, at least to the extent of enabling the duration of incubation to be reduced. Most investigators favor a rather longer period of incubation than the original five minutes. Jørgensen et al[78] compared titration scores of antibodies in different test systems, and determined that the maximum mean score using saline or albumin was attained after 40-60 minutes incubation, whereas the same mean score was reached after only 15-20 minutes when the cells were suspended in LISS. It was also noted by these investigators that mean antiglobulin titration scores were only slightly higher when albumin was added to the test system than when it was not present; and that the mean score showed a sudden decrease when the incubation time was extended beyond 40 minutes in the LISS test procedure. It therefore appears likely that incubation for 15 minutes is inadequate for maximum sensitivity in conventional indirect antiglobulin test procedures, and that the main advantage of the LISS system is to enable satisfactory antibody uptake to be achieved within this time. It may be a disadvantage, however, that sensitivity has been reported[78] to be impaired if the test is inadvertently incubated for longer than the optimum. Voak et al[79] were unable to confirm a sudden fall in titration scores when LISS tests were incubated for longer than 40 minutes, but agreed that their experiments had shown incubation for 20 minutes at low ionic strength to be for all practical purposes as reliable as incubation for 90 minutes in conventional saline-antiglobulin tests.

Summation and Conclusion

For greater sensitivity and consistent reliability in the detection of unexpected blood group antibodies it is possible, as Rosenfield and his colleagues[67] suggested, that instrumentation should be the long-term goal, with the object of eliminating variables such as human visual acuity and subjective interpretation as the main sources of error. In the meantime, the selection of compatible blood for transfusion must continue to depend largely on the broad-range sensitivity of the indirect antiglobulin test, whether incubation is carried out at normal ionic strength (preferably for a somewhat longer period than is common at present) or at low ionic strength for 15-20 minutes. If the use of potentiators is to give meaningful additional confidence through the promotion of direct agglutination by some immune antibodies, the agent used should be chosen on the basis of proven effectiveness, and employed by a technique that provides reasonable expectation of consistent reliability, rather than convenience of application. The current most widely used technique with bovine albumin provides acceptable sensitivity only if polymerized albumin is used. An alternative would be to modify the test procedure in such a way as to eliminate from the test system the aqueous fluid in which the red cell component is suspended.

In the area of red cell typing, high-protein antisera containing macromolecular additives have shown acceptable reliability for the detection of Rh antigens for many years, subject only to the minor inconvenience of the control test needed to detect spontaneous agglutination. It would be difficult to sacrifice the accustomed strong reactions given by this kind of antiserum, even though chemical modification of the IgG molecule can be utilized to prepare antiserums that contain a lower concentration of bovine albumin that agglutinate antigen-positive red cells without macromolecular additives and do not promote the spontaneous agglutination of immunoglobulin-coated red cells. The exclusive use of these reagents, however, may be attended by failure to recognize some weak variant antigens, as a low-protein test system is inherently less sensitive than a potentiated high-protein one. Accordingly, any advantage gained through the diminished incidence of false positives caused by spontaneous agglutination must be balanced against some inevitable loss of sensitivity in detecting weakly expressed antigens.

References

1. Landsteiner K. Über Agglutinationserscheinungen normalen menschlichen Blutes. Wien Klin Wschr 1901;14:1132-4.
2. Landsteiner K, Levine P. A new agglutinable factor differentiating individual human bloods. Proc Soc Exp Biol 1927;24:600-2.
3. Landsteiner K, Levine P. Further observations on individual differences of human blood. Proc Soc Exp Biol 1927;24:941-2.
4. Landsteiner K, Wiener AS. A agglutinable factor in human blood recognized by immune sera for rhesus blood. Proc Soc Exp Biol 1940;43:223.
5. Levine P, Stetson RE. An unusual case of intragroup agglutination. JAMA 1939;113:126-7.
6. Wiener AS, Peters HR. Hemolytic reactions following transfusion of blood of the homologous group, with three cases in which the same agglutinogen was responsible. Ann Intern Med 1940; 13:2306-22.
7. Race RR. An "incomplete" antibody in human serum. Nature 1944;153:771-2.
8. Wiener AS. A new test (blocking test) for Rh sensitization. Proc Soc Exp Biol 1944;56:173-6.
9. Marrack JR. The chemistry of antigens and antibodies. London: HM Stationery Office, 1938.
10. Diamond LK, Abelson NM. The demonstration of anti-Rh agglutinins, an accurate and rapid slide test. J Lab Clin Med 1945; 30:204-12.
11. Wiener AS. Conglutination test for Rh sensitization. J Lab Clin Med 1945;30:662-7.
12. Diamond LK, Abelson NM. The demonstration of Rh sensitization: evaluations of tests for Rh antibodies. J Lab Clin Med 1945; 30:668-74.
13. Diamond LK, Denton RL. Rh agglutination in various media with particular reference to the value of albumin. J Lab Clin Med 1945; 30:821-30.
14. Cameron JW, Diamond LK. Chemical, clinical and immunological studies on the products of human plasma fractionation. XXIX. Serum albumin as a diluent for Rh typing reagents. J Clin Invest 1945;24:793-801.

15. Wiener AS, Hurst JG, Sonn-Gordon EB. Studies on the conglutination reaction with special reference to the nature of conglutinin. J Exp Med 1947;86:267-84.
16. Bordet J, Streng O. Le phénomène d'absorption et la conglutinine du sérum de boeuf. Zbl Bakt 1909;49:260.
17. Wiener AS. The solution of certain fundamental immunological problems by studies on Rh sensitization. Ann Allerg 1952; 10:535-54.
18. Wiener AS, Hurst JG, Handman L. Emploi de gélatine et d'autres produits de remplacement pour le titrage des anticorps Rh univalents par la réaction de conglutination. Rev Hémat 1948;3:3-12.
19. Levine P. The present status of the Rh factor. Am J Clin Pathol 1946;16:597-620.
20. Grubb R. Dextran as a medium for the demonstration of incomplete anti-Rh agglutinins. J Clin Pathol 1949;2:223-4.
21. Jones AR. Dextran as a diluent for univalent antibodies. Nature 1950;165:118-9.
22. McNeil C, Trentelman EF. Detection of antibodies by polyvinylpyrrolidone (PVP). Am J Clin Pathol 1952;22:77-82.
23. Hirszfeld L, Dubiski S. Untersuchungen über die Struktur der inkompletten Antikörper. Schweiz Zeitschr Path Bakt 1954;10:535.
24. Pollack W, Hager HJ, Reckel R, Toren DA, Singher DA. A study of the forces involved in the second stage of hemagglutination. Transfusion 1965;5:158-83.
25. Wiener AS, Katz L. Studies on the use of enzyme-treated red cells on tests for Rh sensitization. J Immunol 1951;66:51-66.
26. Hughes-Jones NC, Gardner B. Telford R. The effect of ficin on the reaction between anti-D and red cells. Vox Sang 1964;9:175-82.
27. Hummel K. Der Vorgang der Haemagglutination durch komplette und inkomplette Antikörper. Deutsch Gesund 1964;20:321.
28. Greenwalt TJ, Steane EA. Quantitative hemagglutination. VI: Relationship of sialic acid content of red cells and aggregation by Polybrene,® protamine and poly-L-lysine. Br J Haematol 1973; 25:227-37.
29. Steane EA. Thermodynamic studies of erythrocyte antigen-antibody interaction and the modulation of this phenomenon by partial enzymatic digestion of the cell membrane, PhD dissertation, Washington, DC: The George Washington University, 1974.
30. Steane EA, Greenwalt TJ. Red cell agglutination. Experimental evidence suggesting an important role for vicinal water. In: Mohn JF, Plunkett RW, Cunningham RK, Lambert RM, eds. Human blood groups, Basel: Karger, 1977:36-43.

31. Good W, Wood JE. The hydration effect of alkali metal and halide ions on the Rh-anti-Rh system. Immunology 1971;20:37-42.

32. Good W, Wood JE. The hydrational effect of alkaline-earth chlorides and selected nonelectrolytes on the Rh-anti-Rh system. Immunology 1971;21:617-22.

33. Good W, Wood JE. Hydrational aspects of A-anti-A and B-anti-B interactions. Immunology 1972;23:423-7.

34. Hughes-Jones NC, Gardner B, Telford R. Studies on the reaction between blood-group antibody anti-D and erythrocytes. Biochem J 1963;88:435-40.

35. Steane EA. The physical chemistry of hemagglutination. In: Walker RH, ed. A seminar on polymorphisms in human blood. Washington, DC: American Association of Blood Banks, 1975: 105-27.

36. Schroeder V. Physical-chemical processes in isohaemagglutination. Pfluger Arch Gesund Physiol 1926;215:32.

37. Hughes-Jones NC, Gardner B. The Kell system studies with radioactively-labelled anti-K. Vox Sang 1971;21:154-8.

38. Hughes-Jones NC, Gardner B, Lincoln PJ. Observations on the number of available c, D and E antigen sites on red cells. Vox Sang 1971;21:210-6.

39. Stratton F, Renton PH. Practical blood grouping. Springfield: Charles C. Thomas, 1958.

40. Grove-Rasmussen M, Dreisler N, Shaw RS. A serologic study of 8 samples of anti-Kell serum, with special emphasis on crossmatching technics that will detect incompatibility due to anti-Kell antibodies as well as anti-A, anti-B and Rh antibodies. Am J Clin Pathol 1954;24:1211-19.

41. Stratton F, Rawlinson VI, Gunson HH, Phillips PK. The role of zeta potential in Rh agglutination. Vox Sang 1973;24:273-9.

43. Greenbury CL, Moore DH, Nunn LAC. Reaction of 7S and 19S components of immune rabbit antisera with human group A and AB red cells. Immunology 1963;6:421-33.

44. Voak D, Downie DM. The sensitivity of the Rh-anti-Rh system to ordered water of hydration. Immunology 1974;26:673-5.

45. Brooks DE, Seaman GVF. The effect of neutral polymers on the electrokinetic potential of cells and other charged particles. I. Models for the zeta potential increase. J Colloid Interf Sci 1973; 43:670-86.

46. Jan K-M, Chien S. Role of surface charge in red blood cell interactions. J Gen Physiol 1973;61:638-54.

47. Jones GE. Intercellular adhesion: modification by dielectric prop-

erties of the medium J Membr Biol 1974;16:297-312.

48. Brooks DE. The effect of neutral polymers on the electrokinetic potentials of cells and other charged particles. IV. Electrostatic effects in dextran-mediated cellular interactions. J Colloid Interf Sci 1973;43:714-26.

49. Jones JM, Kekwick RA, Goldsmith KLG. Influence of polymers on the efficacy of serum albumin as a potentiator of "incomplete" Rh agglutinins. Nature 1969;224:510-11.

50. Oss CJ van, Mohn JF, Cunningham RK. Physicochemical aspects of hemagglutination. In: Mohn JF, Plunkett RW, Cunningham RK, Lambert RM, eds. Human blood groups, Basel: Karger 1974:56-64.

51. Oss CJ van, Mohn JF, Cunningham RK. Influence of various physicochemical factors on hemagglutination. Vox Sang 1978; 34:351-61.

52. Oss CJ van, Good RJ, Neumann AN. The connection of interfacial free energies and surface potentials with phagocytosis and cellular adhesiveness. J Electroanal Chem 1971;37:387-91.

53. Salsbury AJ, Clark JA. Surface charges in red blood cells undergoing agglutination. Rev Franc Etud Clin Biol 1967;12:981-5.

54. Oss CJ van, Mohn JF. Scanning electron microscopy of red cell agglutination. Vox Sang 1970;19:432-43.

55. Coombs RRA, Mourant AE, Race RR. A new test for the detection of weak and "incomplete" antibodies. Brit J Exp Path 1945; 26:255-66.

56. Stratton F. Rapid Rh typing, a "sandwich" technique. Br Med J 1955;i:201-3.

57. Dunsford I, Bowley CC. Techniques in blood grouping. London: Oliver and Boyd 1955:97.

58. Case J. The albumin layering method for D typing. Vox Sang 1959;4:403-5.

59. Wiener AS, Hurst J. A new sensitive (direct) test for Rh blocking antibodies. Exp Med Surg 1947;5:285-98.

60. Stratton F, Dimond ER. The value of serum and albumin mixture for use in the detection of blood group antigen-antibody reactions. J Clin Pathol 1955;8:218-24.

61. Stroup M, MacIlroy M. Evaluation of the albumin antiglobulin technic in antibody detection. Transfusion 1965;5:184-91.

62. Rosenfield RE, Spitz C, Bar-Shany S, Permoad P, DuCros M. Low ionic concentration to augment hemagglutination for the detection and measurement of serological incompatibility. In: Automation in analytical chemistry (1967 Technicon Symposia). White Plains: Medical Inc., 1968:173.

63. Lalezari P. A new method for the detection of red cell antibodies. In: Automation in analytical chemistry (1967 Technicon Symposia). White Plains: Medical Inc., 1968:169.

64. Lalezari P. A new method for the detection of red blood cell antibodies. Transfusion 1968;5:184-91.

65. Hummel K. Über die Wirkungsweise der Konglutinationsteste zum Nachweis inkompletter Agglutinine. Zbl Bakt Parasit Infekt Krankh Hyg 1951;157:176.

66. Spielmann W. Mitteilung über die Beeinflussung konglutinierender Anti-Rh-Seren durch verschiedene Chemikalien. Z Immunforsch 1954;111:471.

67. Rosenfield RE, Shaikh SH, Innella F, Kaczera Z, Kochwa S. Augmentation of hemagglutination by low ionic conditions. Transfusion 1979;19:499-510.

68. Atchley WA, Bhagavan NV, Masouredis SP. Effect of ionic strength on the reaction between anti-D and D-positive red cells. J Immunol 1964;93:701-12.

69. Elliot M, Bossom W, Dupuy ME, Masouredis SP. Effect of ionic strength on the behavior of red cell isoantibodies. Vox Sang 1964;9:396-414.

70. Hughes-Jones NC, Gardner B, Telford R. The effect of ionic strength on the reaction between anti-D and erythrocytes. Immunology 1965;7:72-81.

71. Hughes-Jones NC, Polley MJ, Telford R. Gardner B, Kleinschmidt G. Optimal conditions for detecting blood group antibodies by the antiglobulin test. Vox Sang 1964;9:385-395.

72. Löw B, Messeter L. Antiglobulin test in low ionic strength salt solution for rapid antibody screening and crossmatching. Vox Sang 1974;26:53-61.

73. Wicker B, Wallas CH. A comparison of low ionic strength saline medium with routine methods for antibody identification. Transfusion 1976;16:469-72.

74. Lincoln PJ, Dodd BE. The use of low ionic strength solution (LISS) in elution experiments and in combination with papain-treated cells for titration of various antibodies, including eluted antibody. Vox Sang 1978;34:221-6.

76. Rock G, Baxter A, Charron M, Jhaveri J. LISS—an effective way to increase blood utilization. Transfusion 1978;18:228-32.

77. Fitzsimmons JM, Morel PA. The effects of red blood cell suspending media on hemagglutination and the antiglobulin test. Transfusion 1979;19:81-5.

78. Jørgensen J, Nielsen M, Nielsen CB, Nørmark J. The influence of

ionic strength, albumin and incubation time on the sensitivity of the indirect Coombs' test. Vox Sang 1979;36:186-91.

79. Voak D, Downie DM, Darnborough J, Haigh T, Fairham SA. Low-ionic strength media for rapid antibody detection: optimum conditions and quality control. Med Lab Technol 1980;37:107-18.

7

Action and Application of Enzymes in Immunohematology

Sandra S. Ellisor, MT (ASCP) SBB

Introduction

ENZYMES HAVE BEEN USED in such food processing as wine and cheese making and leavening of bread as far back as ancient Greek times. Prior to the 20th century, little was known about the nature and function of enzymes. In the 19th century fermentation of wine was attributed to a substance produced by yeast.[1] In 1878, the term "enzyme" was first used for a substance extracted from pancreas which was able to digest proteins. The term comes from the Greek words meaning "in yeast."[1,2] It was not until 1926 that the first enzyme was purified in enough quantity for the chemical nature of the enzyme to be identified. Since that time the structure, kinetics and actions of certain enzymes have been studied intensely.[2] In 1946, Pickles[3] was the first to report the use of enzymes for red blood cell agglutination studies, and in 1950, Porter[4] reported using enzymes to study the structure of antibody molecules.

Enzymes are proteins which are efficient and specific at catalyzing reactions. They accelerate the rate of one type of chemical reaction with one type of compound (or substrate) by factors of at least one million.[5] As with all biological reactions, enzymatic reactions are affected by ionic strength, pH and temperature. Substrate specificity of enzymes is primarily due to the three-dimensional shape of the enzyme reaction site and the shape complementarity of the substrate reaction site. During the enzymatic reaction, noncovalent bonds are formed between the enzyme and substrate which accelerate the making or breaking of covalent bonds within the substrate. The enzyme will then dissociate, unchanged, from the modified substrate.[5] Isolated enzymes can be unstable and may deteriorate during storage.[6]

Sandra S. Ellisor, MT (ASCP) SBB, Director, Reference and Education, American Red Cross Blood Services, Central California Region, San Jose, California.

Classification and Nomenclature

Enzymes may be classified and named according to the chemical nature of the enzyme, the chemical nature of the substrate, or the type of reaction they catalyze. At the recommendation of the International Union of Biochemistry,[7] a systematic classification code number is given to each enzyme based on the reaction catalyzed and the substrate specificity. The six main classes of enzymatic reactions are:

1. Oxidoreductases—catalyze reactions (oxidoreduction) in which hydrogen is transferred.

2. Transferases—catalyze the transfer of a chemical group from a donor compound to an acceptor compound.

3. Hydrolases—catalyze the introduction of elements of water at a specific site in a substrate molecule.

4. Lyases—catalyze nonhydrolytic substrate cleavage with formation of double bonds.

5. Isomerases—catalyze geometric or structural changes within a molecule.

6. Ligases—catalyze the joining of two molecules coupled with hydrolysis of ATP and production of high energy bonds.

A systematic and a common or "trivial" name is also given to each enzyme. As with the classification codes, a systematic name is based on the reaction catalyzed and the substrate specificity. The systematic name indicates the action of an enzyme as exactly as possible, identifies the enzyme precisely, but does not include the source of the enzyme. The common name is sufficiently short for general use, not necessarily systematic, and may be the name originally given to the enzyme.[7] Since, in immunohematology, we are usually interested in identifying the biochemical structure of substances and the activation or inactivation of antigens, the classes of enzymes we most commonly

---

Table 1.—Classes and General Substrate Specificities of Some Hydrolytic Enzymes[7]

Common Names(s)	Substrate(s)
peptidases, proteinases, proteases	peptides, proteins, amino acids
nucleases	nucleic acids
amylases	starch
phosphatases	phosphate esters
lipases	fats, lipids
glycosidases	glucose, carbohydrates

use are hydrolases and, occasionally, transferases. Common names of transferases are formed to include the group being transferred (eg, transaminases transfer amino groups, transglycosidases transfer glucose groups). Hydrolases are commonly named by the addition of "ase" to the substrate (Table 1). The prefixes "exo" or "endo" may be added to the stem word to indicate action of the enzyme on terminal or internal substrate linkages respectively. Other qualifying terms used with the common name usually refer to specific properties of the enzyme reaction site (ie, serine endoproteinase).

Sources

Enzymes are extracted from plants, fungi, bacterial and viral culture filtrates, animal tissues, secretions or body fluids (Tables 2 and 3). Some proteolytic enzymes are available as purified, crystallized products,[8-9] but many proteolytic enzymes are used as crude extracts. These crude extracts often contain contaminating enzymes. Anywhere from two to ten active proteolytic compounds have been found in ficin extracts.[16] Crude extracts of papain can contain papain, chymopapain and papaya peptidase A, while crude trypsin may contain contaminating chymotrypsin. Bromelain, also referred to as bromelin, may have up to four distinct proteolytic components. Bromelase is a crude precursor form of bromelain which contains all of the material extracted from stems of pineapple plants and may contain several proteolytic enzymes as well as acid phosphatase.[17-18] As would be expected, use of crude extracts may lead to variable test results.[19-20]

Reaction Site Characteristics

The four subdivisions of the proteolytic enzymes in Table 3 are based on properties of the enzyme reaction site.[7] Serine proteinases have essential serine and histidine residues in the active site. Thiol proteinases have an essential cysteine in the enzyme active site and activation of the enzyme may be required with a sulfhydryl compound. Carboxyl proteinases have an essential COOH in the enzyme active site and require acidic pH. Metalloproteinases require a specific metal ion in the enzyme active site. Amino acid sequence comparisons of some thiol enzymes near the essential cysteine residue indicate similar sterochemistry of binding sites for ficin, papain and bromelain, while chymopapain is similar to Streptococcal proteinase.[18]

The first prerequisite for the action of a given enzyme is bond or sequence substrate specificity.[15] Substrate specificities for those hydrolytic enzymes that have been used to treat red blood cells for sero-

135

Table 2.—Classification, Common Names, Sources and Immunochemical Studies for Glycosidic Enzymes Used in Immunohematology

Classification	Name(s)	Sources[8-10]	Red Blood Cell Antigen Studies
exoglycosidase	neuraminidase, sialidase, RDE (receptor destroying enzyme)	Vibrio cholerae, Influenza virus, Clostridium perfringens	M, N[10]
	α-N-acetylgalactosaminidase	Charonia lampus liver (marine gastropod)	A[11]
	α-L-fucosidase	bovine epididymis and kidney	H, Le[a], Le[b][11]
	β-galactosidase	bovine liver, Aspergillus niger, Escherichia coli, Jack beans	I[12]
	β-N-acetylhexosaminidase	bovine epididymis, porcine and human placenta	I[12]
	α-D-galactosidase	green coffee beans, Aspergillus niger	B, I[11-12]
	β-N-acetylglucosaminidase	Aspergillus niger, bovine kidney, human placenta, Jack beans	I[12]
endoglycosidase	endo-β-galactosidase	Escherichia freundii	ABH, Ii, Tk[13,14]

Table 3.—Classifications, Names, Sources and pH Optimum for Proteolytic Enzymes Which Have Been Used in Immunohematology

Classification	Name	Sources[7-9]	pH Optimum
serine endoproteinases	chymotrypsin	bovine and porcine pancreas	neutral[15]
	trypsin	bovine and porcine pancreas	neutral[15]
	proteinase K	Tritirachium album (mold)	alkaline[7]
thiol endoproteinases (sulfhydryl enzymes, plant latex enzymes)	papain	papaya latex	neutral[15]
	ficin	ficus latex	neutral[16]
	bromelain	pineapple stem	neutral[16]
carboxyl proteinase	pepsin	porcine stomach mucosa	acidic[15]
metalloproteinases	neutral proteinase	Bacillus subtilis	neutral[7]
	pronase	Streptomyces griseus	neutral[7]

acidic pH < 5
neutral pH 6-7
alkaline pH 8-10

logic testing are listed in Table 4. Trypsin has the most restricted substrate specificity and proteinase K the broadest. However, trypsin has the broadest steric specificity since it will cleave all bonds to the carboxyl group of any arginine or lysine residue in most peptides regardless of adjacent amino acid residues.[15] Neutral proteases (Table 3) hydrolyze mainly peptide bonds involving amino groups of hy-

Table 4.—Amino Acid Substrate Specificities of Hydrolytic Enzymes Commonly Used to Treat Red Blood Cells for Serological Testing[7,21]

Enzyme	Substrates
trypsin	arginine, lysine
Bacillus subtilis neutral proteinase	−leucine > −phenalanine
papain	arginine, lysine, phenylalanine-X- (the bond next but one to the carboxyl group of phenylalanine)
chymotrypsin	tyrosine, tryptophan, phenylalanine, leucine
bromelain	lysine, alanine, tyrosine, glycine
ficin	lysine, alanine, tyrosine, glycine, asparagine, leucine, valine
pronase	bonds adjacent to hydrophobic amino acids
proteinase K	bonds at the carboxyl of aromatic or hydrophobic amino acid residues
neuraminidases	
bacterial	O-acetylated neuraminic acid (C7 or C8); $\alpha2{\to}3$, $\alpha2{\to}4$, $\alpha2{\to}6$, or $\alpha2{\to}8$ ketosidically linked NANA
viral	O-acetylated neuraminic acid (C4, C7 or C8); $\alpha2{\to}3$ ketosidically linked NANA

drophobic amino acid residues while alkaline proteases hydrolyze peptide bonds linking carboxyl groups of hydrophobic amino acid residues.[22] Bacterial neuraminidases have a more limited specificity than viral neuraminidases for O-acetylated neuraminic acid but have a broader specificity at the α ketosidic linkages of NANA.[21] The spacial arrangement of molecular chains can modify the enzymatic reaction even if bond or substrate specificity is present. Enzymes can only cleave bonds that are accessible and can fit the enzyme binding site or those which are flexible enough to move to fit the binding site.[15]

Serologic Uses of Enzymes

Red Cells

In 1946, Pickles[3] first reported agglutination of washed IgG-sensitized red cells upon incubation with a Vibrio cholera broth culture filtrate. Since that time, cell membrane structure and enzyme modification of red cells have been studied extensively. External portions of cellular membranes are composed of proteins and lipids. Carbohydrates may be attached to both, forming glycoproteins or glycolipids.[23] Lipases cleave bonds on components in lipids or glycolipid chains. Since the bilipid layer maintains the integrity of cell membranes, the action of lipases may cause lysis of the cells. Glycosidic enzymes cleave bonds in carbohydrate chains on glycoproteins or glycolipids without affecting the integrity of the cell membrane. Proteolytic enzymes cleave bonds in appropriate amino acid chains of membrane bound proteins or glycoproteins. Progressive proteolytic enzyme modification of red cells can result in the following general serologic stages: (1) enhanced reactivity with some alloantibodies; (2) denaturation of certain red cell antigens; (3) agglutination with all "alloantibody-free" sera; (4) agglutination in saline; and, eventually, (5) hemolysis.[6,24] The physical effects of mild treatment of red cells with trypsin was studied by Ponder.[25] He reported a significant decrease in the electrophoretic mobility of trypsin-treated red cells but only slight loss of tonicity, decrease in density, and increase in red cell volume, osmotic and mechanical fragility. There was no consistent alteration in red cell shape or shape transformation when viewed through a light microscope. Van Oss and Mohn[26] studied papain-treated red cells using a scanning electron microscope and found the red cells had lost tonicity, become deformed, and their surface had become "thready and corrugated." The decrease in electrophoretic mobility of enzyme treated red cells is due to removal of N-acetyl neuraminic acid (NANA), which is a carbohydrate, the only sialic acid found on the red cell membrane, and the principal charged component of the red cell membrane.[27]

The enzymes most often used in serologic investigations are the proteolytic enzymes trypsin, ficin, papain, and bromelain, and the glycosidic enzyme neuraminidase. Neuraminidase removes terminal NANA residues from glycoproteins and glycolipids on the red cell membrane while proteolytic enzymes cleave proteins and sialoglycoproteins (NANA + glucoses + proteins) from the red cell surface.[27-28] Mild enzyme treatment of red cells may result in the following serologic effects: (1) exposure of "new" antigens; (2) antigen denaturation, and (3) antibody reactivity enhancement.

"New" Antigens

"New" antigens may be either antigens that are not normally expressed on the red cell membrane (cryptantigens) or antigens that are present on the red cell membrane but are not as accessible to the corresponding antibody (latent antigens). Enzymatic removal of carbohydrates or sialoglycoproteins (SGPs) could result in "uncovering" or altering the configuration of cryptantigens, latent antigens or both.[29-35] As a generalization, glycosidic enzymes tend to expose cryptantigens and small numbers of latent antigens while proteolytic enzymes tend to expose large numbers of latent antigens. Table 5 lists the "new" antigens exposed by hydrolytic enzymes.

Table 5.—"New" Antigens Exposed on Red Cell Membranes by Treatment with Hydrolytic Enzymes

Type	Antigen(s)	Enzyme
cryptantigens	T	neuraminidase[29]
	T_k	endo-β-galactosidase[30]
latent antigens	Rh, I, i	{ neuraminidase[31-32] trypsin, ficin, papain and bromelain[32-35]

The cryptantigen T is composed of the disaccharide galactose ($\beta 1 \rightarrow 3$) N-acetyl-galactosamine.[36] This disaccharide is a sialiated component of the alkali-labile tetrasaccharides found attached to serine and threonine residues on both the MN and Ss SGPs (Fig 1) as well as the carbohydrate component of some globosides (Fig 2). Neuraminidase removes the terminal NANA from these substrates exposing this disaccharide and "T activating" the red cells.

N-acetyl-glucosamine appears to be the immunodominant sugar responsible for expression of the T_k antigen.[30] Endo-β-galactosidase treatment of red cells exposes this sugar within the ABH and I oligosaccharides (Fig 2) found on glycoproteins and glycolipids and other glycosphingolipids and results in exposure of the T_k antigen.

Vicia graminea detects galactose ($\beta 1 \rightarrow 3$) N-acetyl-galactosamine as well as the linkages to serine or threonine residues on the NH_2 terminal portion of untreated N SGPs, but conformationally does not

140

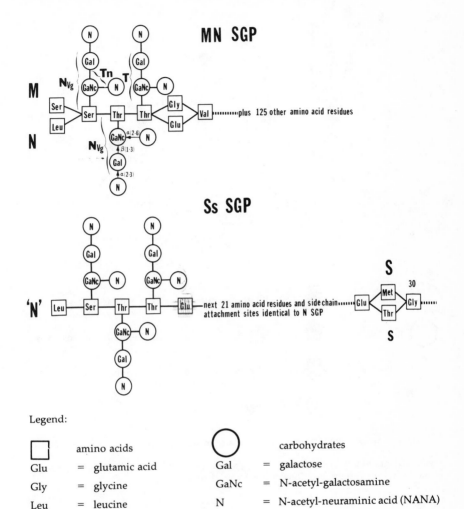

Legend:

☐   amino acids

Glu   =   glutamic acid

Gly   =   glycine

Leu   =   leucine

Met   =   methionine

Thr   =   threonine

Ser   =   serine

Val   =   valine

◯   carbohydrates

Gal   =   galactose

GaNc   =   N-acetyl-galactosamine

N   =   N-acetyl-neuraminic acid (NANA)

Fig 1.—Diagrammatic representation of biochemical structure of M,N,S,s,'N',T,Tn and N_{Vg} antigens.[36-38]

141

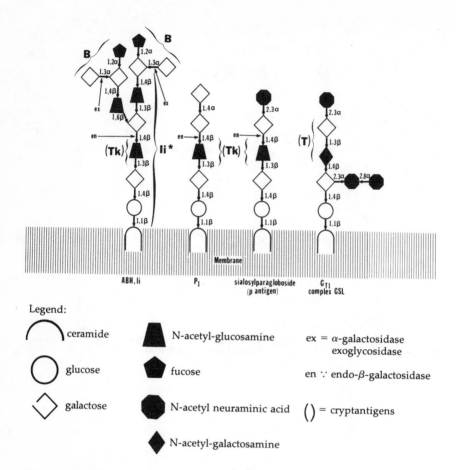

Legend:

⌢ ceramide   ◣ N-acetyl-glucosamine   ex = α-galactosidase
exoglycosidase

◯ glucose   ⬠ fucose   en ∵ endo-β-galactosidase

◇ galactose   ⬤ N-acetyl neuraminic acid   ( ) = cryptantigens

◆ N-acetyl-galactosamine

*i antigen is unbranched chains; I antigen is branched chains.

Fig 2.—Diagrammatic representation of glycosphingolipids (GSLs) in the red cell membrane including antigen locations and enzyme cleavage sites.[39-41]

have access to these internal regions on untreated M SGPs[42] (Fig 1). Neuraminidase removal of NANA exposes crypt N_{Vg} receptors within the alkali labile tetrasaccharide on the NH_2 terminal portion of M SGP.

Removal of NANA slightly reduces steric hindrance and results in exposure of small quantities of latent Rh, I and i antigens on neuraminidase treated red cells.[31-32] Exposure of more latent Rh, I and i antigens have been demonstrated using proteolytic enzymes because removal of the larger SGP fragments results in a greater reduction in steric hindrance.[32-35]

Antigen Denaturation

Enzymatic removal of carbohydrates or SGP may reduce the reactivity of an antibody with its corresponding antigen. This has been termed antigen destruction, inactivation, or denaturation at various times during the history of serologic investigation. Antigen destruction would occur if the antigen combining sites were removed due to cleavage from the red cell membrane.[29] In many cases, the use of endoenzymes (endoproteases and endoglycosidases) results in total antigen destruction by this mechanism. Antigen inactivation or denaturation could also occur if a constituent necessary for the conformational specificity of the antigen combining site were removed or altered.[29] Denaturation of antigens by this mechanism occurs in many instances using exoglycosidases, but presumably may also occur using the endoenzymes.

Denaturation of red cell antigens using hydrolytic enzymes has been extensively studied. Table 6 lists the reported effects of many hydrolytic enzymes on human red cell antigens. Numerous discrepancies can be observed. Some are probably attributable to variations in the type and amounts of contaminating enzymes found in crude enzyme extracts. Judson and Anstee reported the denaturation of Fy^a and Kell antigens by crude trypsin preparation was due to contaminating chymotrypsin since crystallized trypsin did not denature either of these antigens.[20] They also demonstrated that Kell antigens could be denatured by the action of trypsin and chymotrypsin simultaneously or sequentially, but not separately.

Discrepancies in antigen denaturation may also be due to variations in standardization of enzyme modification procedures.[20,68] Using a spectrophotometric method for detecting enzyme activity, Lambert et al[92] reported proteolytic activity in 1% w/v solutions of ficin, bromelain and papain to be 245, 86 and 50 units/cm, respectively. Using a modification of this procedure, Draper[93] not only found variations in enzyme activity between types of crude enzyme preparations, but also between different commercial sources of each crude enzyme (213-165, 323-150, 650-400, 490-160 units/ml for ficin, bromelain, papain and trypsin respectively). In serologic studies by Issitt,[94] denaturation of the M, N, S, Fy^a, and Fy^b antigens were obtained using crude extracts of ficin, papain, bromelain and trypsin if the enzymes were used under optimum conditions of temperature, concentration, pH and activation time. In comparison, trypsin had to be used at ten times greater concentrations (% w/v) and for four times longer than ficin. This correlates with the data from Steane[95] on efficiency of NANA removal from red cell membranes in the order ficin > papain > brome-

Table 6.—Effect of Specific Hydrolytic

Blood Group System	Antigens	Unspecified Protease	Trypsin—Unknown Purity	Crude Trypsin	Crystalline Trypsin	Crystalline Chymotrypsin	Trypsin → Chymotrypsin or Chymotrypsin → Trypsin
ABH I	Unspecified		+ or ↑ (43-45) ↑ (47)	↑ (32)	↑ (46)		
	I^F	+ (50)					
	I^D	↑ (50)					
i		↑ (50)		↑ (32)			
Sp_1 Pr				↓ (51)			
	Pr_{1-3} Pr_a		0 (53)				
Gd Sa Fl Lud							
Indian	In^a In^b	0 (56)	↓ or0(55)				
T Tn Tk			↓ (59)		+ (60)		
En^a							
	En^aTS		0 (62)				
	En^aFS		+ (62)				
	En^aFR		+ (62)				
Wright	Wr^a Wr^b						
MNSs	Unspecified M		↓ (45)				
	$\neq M_{Hum}$		0 (44,64) ↓ (65)	0 (46) ↓ (64)	0 (20,66) ↑ (46)	↓ (20)+(66)	
	$\neq M_{Rab}$		0 (44)		+ or0(20)0(66,68)	+ (20,66,68)	
	Unspecified N		↓ (45)				
	$\neq N_{Hum}$		↓ (65)	0 (46)	↑ (46)0or+(66)	+ (66)	
	$\neq N_{Rab}$		0 (44)		↓ (20)+(66)0(68)	+ (20,66,68)	
	$\neq N_{Vg}$				+ (20,66)	+ (24,66)	
	N_{Form}						
	'N'		↑ (45,65)		+ or ↑ (66) ↑ (70)	0 (66,70)	
	S		↑ (44)0(68)	0 (46)+(64)	↑ (46)+(20,66,68)	+ or ↓ (20)0(66,68)	
	s			+ (64)	+ (20,66)	+ (20)0(66)	
	U						
	M_1						
	M_g		0 (43,72)				
	Cl^a		0 (73)				
	Je^a		0 (74)				
	Ny^a						

Enzymes on Human Red Cell Antigens*

Papain	Ficin	Bromelain	Neutral Proteinase	Pronase	Proteinase K	Neuraminidase	Endo-β-galactosidase	Phospholipase A₂ or C
↑ (32,48)	↑ (32,47)	↑ (32)			↑ (48)	↑ (32) + (50) ↑ (39)	↓ (14) ↓ or0(14,49)	
↑ (32,48)	↑ (32)	↑ (32)			↑ (48)	↑ (32,50)	0 (14)	
0 (51)	0 (51)	↓ (51)						
0 (52) 0 (53) + (52) ↓ (50) + (50) ↓ (50)	0 (53)	0 (53)			0 (48)	0 (52) + (53) 0 (52) 0 (50) 0 (50) 0 (50)		
↓ or0(54,55)		↓ or0(55)				↓ or0(55)		
+, ↓ or0(57) 0 (57,59)	↓ or0(57)0(58) 0 (57) ↓ (59) ↑ (58)					+ (59-60) + (58) + (61)	+ (58) + (30)	
0 (62) 0 (62) + (62)	0 (62) 0 (62) + (62) ↑ (61) ↓ (61)					+ (61) + (61)		
+ (48,63) ↓ (65) 0 (68)	+ (63) 0 (65,67) ↓ (64,65) 0 (68)	↓ (48)+(63) + (63) ↓ (48,64) 0 (68)	+ (63)	0 (20) 0 (20)	+ (48)	0 (43)0,+or ↑ (62) 0 (62)		
+ (48,63) ↓ (65) 0 (68)	+ (63) ↓ (65) 0 (68) 0 (67)	↓ (48)+(63) 0 (68)	+ (63)	0 (20) 0 (67)	+ (48)	0 , ↓ or+(62)0(43) 0 , ↓ or+(62) 0 (43) ↑ (62) 0 (62)		
↓ (65)	↑ or+(65)							
+ or0(64)0(68,71) 0 (64,71)	+ (64)0(67,68) 0 (64)+(67) ↑ (67)	+ or0(64)0(68) 0 (64)	0 (63) 0 (63)	0 (20,71) 0 (20,71)		+ (29) + (29)		
0 (69) 0 (43) 0 (73) 0 (74) 0 (75)	0 (69) 0 (73) 0 (74)	 0 (73) 0 (74)				+ or ↑ (62) + (43)0or+(62)		

Table 6.—Effect of Specific Hydrolytic

Blood Group System	Antigens	Unspecified Protease	Trypsin— Unknown Purity	Crude Trypsin	Crystalline Trypsin	Crystalline Chymotrypsin	Trypsin → Chymotrypsin or Chymotrypsin → Trypsin
Mi^a	Mi^a V^w Hut Mur Hil Anek Raddon Lane		0 (72) +(72) +(72) +(72)		+(76) 0 (76) 0 (76) +(76) ↑(76) ↑(76) +(76) ↑(76)		
Duffy	Fy^a Fy^b		0 (44,45,68) ↑(78) 0 (78)	+(64)	+(20,68)	0 or ↓ (20)0(68)	
Kell	K k Js^b Kp^b		0 (68)+(44,45) +(44)	0 (20)+(64) +(64) +(64)	+(20) ↑(68)	+(20)	0 (20)
Kidd	Jk^a Jk^b						
Lutheran	Lu^a Lu^b		+(45)0(68)	0 (64)	0 (20,68)	0 (20,68)	
Xg^a Chido Rodgers Cartwright John-Milton-Hagen York	Ch^a Rg^a Yt^a Yt^b JMH Yk^a	↓ (82) + or ↑ (85)	0 (80,81) 0 (68+(85) 0 (87)		↑ (68)	0 (68)	
Scianna Rh	SC1 D,c,e		↑ (45)	↑ (46)	0 (90) ↑ (46)		

+ = unaffected
0 = denatured
↑ = enhanced reactivity
↓ = decreased reactivity

* For the blood group system to be mentioned in this table, at least one of these enzymes has been reported to depress or denature one of the system antigens. Except where noted, the studies were performed using intact human red cells.
** red cell stroma
≠ Hum = human
Rab = rabbit
Vg = Vicia graminea
Form = formaldehyde

Enzymes on Human Red Cell Antigens* (continued)

Papain	Ficin	Bromelain	Neutral Proteinase	Pronase	Proteinase K	Neuraminidase	Endo-β-galactosidase	Phospholipase A₂ or C
0 (77)						+ (62) + or ↑ (62) + or ↑ (62)		
+ (78) ↓ (48,71)0(64,68) 0 (78,79)	0 (64,67,68,78) 0 (67,78)	↓ (48)0(64,68,78) 0 (78)	0 (63)	0 (20,71)	↓ (48)	+ (29)		
↓ (48) + (64,68) ↓ (48) ↑ (68) + (64) + (64) 0 (71)	+ (64,68) + (64) + (64)	↓ (48)+ (64,68) ↓ (48) + (64) + (64)		+ or0(20) ↑ (71) 0 (71)	↓ (48) ↓ (48)	+ (29) + (29)		
↓ (71) ↑ (68) + (68)				0 (71)		+ (29)		
0 (71) + (64,68)	+ or0(64) + (68)	+ or0(64) + (68)		0 (20,71)		+ or0(29) + or0(29)		
0 (80,81) 0 (84) 0 (68,86) ↑ (85)	0 (80,81) 0 or ↓ (83) 0 (84)0or ↓ (83) 0 (68) ↑ (85) 0 (83) 0 (88)+(89)0, ↓ or+(83)	0 (80,81)		0 (81)		+ (81)		
↑ (90) ↑ (68)	↑ (90) ↑ (68)	↑ (68)			↑ (48)	↑ (31)		0 (91)**

lain > trypsin. However, in the study by Draper, one-tenth the concentration (units/ml) of bromelain was required to denature the Fy^a antigen as compared to ficin or papain.[93] This might lead to the conclusion that the Fy^a antigen is on proteins other than those that carry large quantities of NANA.

Enzymatic effects on the MNSs blood group system antigens is much easier to understand since the biochemical structures of the MN SGP and Ss SGP have been determined (Fig 1) and the reaction sites of some of the enzymes on the SGPs have been identified (Fig 3). M and N antigen activity is on the MN SGP external to the red cell membrane (NH_2 portion) and within the terminal eight amino acid residues, three of which have alkali labile tetrasaccharides attached.[42] The first 26 amino acid residues and tetrasaccharide side chain attachment sites of the Ss SGP are identical to those found in the N SGP (Fig 1), and the terminal five amino acid residues of the Ss SGP are termed the 'N' (N quotes) antigen. The polymorphism in amino acid residues determining the S and s antigenic determinants is found at the 29th residue of the Ss SGP[99] (Fig 1). However, the antigen activity of both S and s may be influenced by glutamate residues at positions 28 and/or 31 and possibly by the α-linked N-acetyl galactosamine residue on the threonine at position 25. Tables 7 and 8 show the potential enzyme active sites of the proteolytic enzymes on the MN and Ss SGPs if the amino acid substrate specificity is taken into account without considering the sterochemical specificity. The actual enzyme active sites on SGPs extracted from red cell membranes or as demonstrated using intact red cells is shown in Fig 3.

Trypsin reaction sites have been studied more extensively than the other enzymes. The portion of the MN SGP external to the red cell membrane has potential trypsin sensitive sites available at six amino acid residues (Table 7). Trypsin digestion of MN SGP extracts occurs at amino acid residues at positions 30, 39 and 61,[96] while trypsin-sensitive sites on MN SGP of intact red cells occurs proximal to the 25th amino acid residue, presumably at the 30th and 39th residues.[36] The Ss SGP has potential trypsin sensitive sites at amino acid residues number 18 and 35 (Table 8) and trypsin digestion has been reported at both these residues using extracted Ss SGP.[98-99] However, membrane-bound Ss SGP is very trypsin resistant since the 'N' antigen is not denatured by trypsin treatment of intact red cells[66,70] and tryptic glyco-peptides obtained from digestion of intact red cells do not inhibit anti-S or -s sera.[99] It would appear that the trypsin-sensitive sites of membrane bound Ss SGP is either inaccessible or inflexible and unable to move to fit the enzyme-binding site. Tomita and Marchesi[96] have

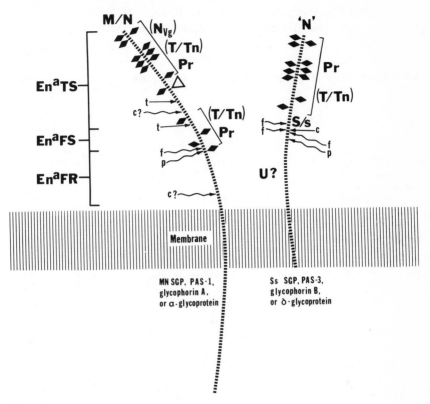

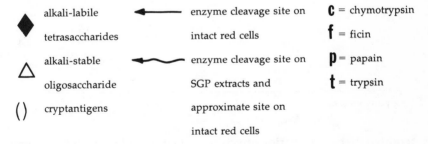

Legend:

◆ alkali-labile tetrasaccharides	⬅— enzyme cleavage site on intact red cells	**C** = chymotrypsin **f** = ficin
△ alkali-stable oligosaccharide	⬳ enzyme cleavage site on SGP extracts and	**p** = papain **t** = trypsin
( ) cryptantigens	approximate site on intact red cells	

Fig 3.—Diagrammatic representation of M/N and S/s sialoglycoproteins in the red cell membrane including antigen locations and enzyme cleavage sites.[36,38,62,96-99]

Table 7.—Potential Amino Acid Residue Reaction Sites
on the MN SGP for Hydrolytic Enzymes[90, 98]

| | | Enzyme | | | |
Chymotrypsin	Trypsin	Papain	Bromelain	Ficin	Pronase
			5*	5*	
				6	6
			7	7	7
					8
				16	16
	18	18	18	18	
20			20	20	
					21
				26	
	30	30	30	30	
	31	31			
34			34	34	
			35	35	35
			36	36	36
					38
	39	39			
			40	40	40
				43	43
					46
				48	48
	49	49			
				51	51
52			52	52	
					53
					54
			59	59	
61	61	61			
				62	62
64				64	64
			65	65	65
68					68
		69			

* if glycine present

reported that glycosylation affects the sensitivity of proteolytic enzyme digestion. Removal of sialic acid from MN SGP extracts and subsequent trypsin treatment resulted in cleavage at an additional amino acid site, residue number 18. Dahr et al[38] also noted additional enzyme cleavage sites on the Ss SGP when using fragments desialyated by neuraminidase.

Chymotrypsin is the other enzyme that has been used extensively in sequencing investigations of extracted SGPs. The external portion of the MN SGP has potential chymotrypsin reaction sites at five amino acid residues (Table 7). Tomita and Marchesi[96] found chymotrypsin cleavage sites on the extracted MN SGP only at amino acid residues number 34 and 64. The actual cleavage site on intact red cells has not been determined, but the membrane bound MN SGP appears resistant to chymotrypsin treatment since the M and N antigens are either not affected[20,66,68] or only slightly depressed[20] on chymotrypsin-treated red cells. The external portion of the Ss SGP that has been characterized has potential chymotrypsin cleavage sites at amino acid residues number 20 and 32. Chymotrypsin has been reported to cleave the Ss SGP only at amino acid residue number 32 on extracted SGP[98] and intact red cells.[38] Serologically, chymotryptic glycopeptides obtained from digestion of appropriate phenotype intact red cells have been found to inhibit both anti-S and -s sera[97] and the S and s antigens on chymotrypsin-treated red cells have been reported to be depressed or denatured.[20,66,68]

No exact enzyme cleavage sites on extracted SGPs or intact red blood cells have been reported for ficin, papain, bromelain or pronase. Anstee[36] approximates enzyme reaction sites for papain and ficin

Table 8.—Potential Amino Acid Residue Reaction Sites on the Ss SGP for Hydrolytic Enzymes[98,99]

| | | Enzyme | | | |
Chymotrypsin	Trypsin	Papain	Bromelain	Ficin	Pronase
				6	6
			7	7	7
					8
				16	16
	18	18	18	18	
20			20	20	
					21
				26	
			27	27	
					29*
			30	30	
32				32	32
				33	33
	35	35			

*if methionine present

below the trypsin reaction sites on the MN SGP; and chymotrypsin, papain and ficin cleavage sites below the 29th amino acid residue (the S or s amino acid determinant) on the Ss SGP.

Serologically, an antigen that is suspected of being carried on either the MN SGP or the Ss SGP can be defined as an MN SGP borne antigen if the reactivity is denatured by trypsin treatment of the red cells.[62] The M and N antigens on the MN SGP will be destroyed by pretreatment[100] of antigen-positive red cells with the proteolytic enzymes trypsin, chymotrypsin, ficin, papain, bromelain and pronase due to cleavage of the immunodominant determinant found within the first eight amino acid residues. If an anti-N antibody reacts with trypsin-treated MM, MN or NN red cells, it will be reacting with the 'N' antigen found on the trypsin resistant Ss SGP.[62,65] The 'N', S and s antigens have been reported as either unaffected[20,64,66,68] or denatured[20,46,64,66,68] by treatment with the proteolytic enzymes chymotrypsin, ficin, papain and bromelain. Pronase consistently denatures the S and s antigens.[20,67] This suggests that, except for chymotrypsin,[20] the other proteolytic enzyme reaction sites on membrane bound MN SGP are readily accessible; while only the pronase reaction site is readily accessible on the Ss SGP. However, Issitt[62,94] reports that if the other proteolytic enzymes are used in high concentration for a long time, these less accessible enzyme reaction sites on the Ss SGP will be affected, resulting in depression or denaturation of the S and s antigens.

Other antigens carried on MN and Ss SGP will be depressed or denatured by proteolytic enzyme treatment of red cells (Fig 3). The cryptantigens T and Tn are found on or within the alkali labile tetrasaccharides (Fig 1) attached to both the MN and Ss SGPs.[36,101] Since the Ss SGP is trypsin resistant, trypsin treatment of red cells can reduce but should not totally destroy T or Tn antigens.[36,59-60] Both T and Tn antigens are denatured by treatment with papain and ficin.[57-58] T antigen is more resistant to denaturation by proteolytic enzymes because alternative sources of T antigen are available on the proteolytic enzyme resistant gangliosides[36] (Fig 2).

Three different specificities of anti-En[a] antibodies have been defined by their reactivity with different types of enzyme-modified red cells[62] (Fig 3). Anti-En[a]TS does not react with trypsin-, ficin- or papain-treated red cells. Anti-En[a]FS reacts with trypsin-treated red cells but does not react with ficin- or papain-treated red cells. The third antibody specificity, anti-En[a]FR reacts with trypsin-, papain- and ficin-treated red cells[62] and therefore must recognize a portion of the MN SGP on the proteolytic enzyme resistant fragment.

Neuraminidase inactivation of M and N antigens occurs due to change in configuration of the antigen site and not because of antigen site cleavage.[42] Neuraminidase removes terminal NANA from residues found on SGPs and other structures on the red cell membrane. Conformational changes in the M or N antigen-combining sites may occur due to the removal of NANA from the second, third, and fourth amino acid residues on the MN SGP (Fig 1). These changes can abolish or diminish the agglutination of antigen-positive red cells by some examples of anti-M or anti-N antibodies.[62] Antibodies that do not react with neuraminidase treated antigen positive red cells are recognizing "NANA dependent" M or N antigen structures while those antibodies that will react with neuraminidase desialized antigen positive red cells are primarily recognizing portions of the amino acid chain and are "NANA independent" M or N antigen structures.

A number of cold autoagglutinins have been reported that are directed against neuraminidase labile red cell antigens. It is still unclear whether neuraminidase denatures these antigens by cleavage of the antigen sites or by changes in the conformation of the antigen sites due to the removal of NANA.[52] The neuraminidase labile antigens Pr_1, Pr_2, and Pr_3 are found predominately on the MN and Ss SGPs since papain treatment totally denatures these antigens.[50] Many of these antibodies have been found to be inhibited by solutions of NANA. The neuraminidase labile antigens Gd and Fl antigens are not affected by papain treatment of red cells.[50,52] Anti-Gd has been found to be inhibited by human gangliosides and is considered a NANA dependent glycolipid antigen.[52] Fl could either be on a protease resistant glycoprotein or might also be a ganglioside structure. Sa and Lud-type neuraminidase labile antigens are only partially denatured by papain.[50] These antigens appear to be found on both the MN and Ss SGPs as well as either protease resistant glycoproteins or glycolipid structures.

The biochemistry of the other blood groups system antigens that are depressed or denatured by proteolytic enzymes has not been defined. At this time, we can only use the serologic data and the general biochemical data to speculate on the position of these antigens on external red cell membrane structures.

Using different isolation techniques, two groups of investigators have reported isolation of Duffy antigens.[102-103] After solubilization using sodium dodecyl sulfate (SDS) and polyacrylamide gel electrophoresis (PAGE), both have reported association of Fy^a antigens with a number of different molecular weight proteins. Some of these proteins have a similar migration mobility to band 3, while others are similar to the MN SGP. Serologically, Fy^a antigen is trypsin and neuraminidase resistant, but chymotrypsin, papain, ficin, bromelain, pronase, and proteinase K sensitive (Table 6). These results would indicate that the Fy[a] antigen is NANA independent and not present on the trypsin sensitive portion of the MN SGP. Duffy antigens of "normal" strength[104] on En(a-) red cells, which lack the MN SGP,[62] offers further evidence that Duffy antigens are not present on the MN SGP. Association of Fy[a] with band 3 could be supported by the evidence that there are chymotrypsin sites but no trypsin-sensitive sites on the portion of band 3 external to the red cell membrane.[105]

The biochemistry of Kell blood group antigens is also unknown at this time, and enzymes should prove to be useful tools in elucidation of their structure. The antigens are neuraminidase and, generally, proteolytic enzyme resistant (Table 6). The fact that Kell antigens are denatured by treatment with trypsin and chymotrypsin either simultaneously or sequentially indicates that cleavage of peptide bonds adjacent to both basic and aromatic amino acid residues is necessary for Kell antigen denaturation.[20] Kell antigens can also be denatured by proteolytic enzymes if a high concentration of a sulfhydryl compound is added to the enzymes.[106] This would seem to indicate that access by these enzymes to amino acid substrate residues on the Kell antigens is blocked by the configuration or flexibility of the reaction site due to the presence of a disulfide bond. Further evidence for the association of disulfide bonds in the structure of Kell system antigens is the evidence that the sulfhydryl compound 2-aminoethylisothiouronium bromide (AET) inactivates all autosomal antigens in the Kell system.[107]

Serologically, Lu[a] has been reported to be denatured by proteolytic enzymes while both Lu[a] and Lu[b] antigens are sensitive to neuraminidase from Influenza virus but resistant to neuraminidase from Vibrio cholerae (Table 6). This would seem to indicate that Lutheran antigens are NANA dependent and are located on enzyme sensitive portions of polypeptide chains. However, this interpretation is not consistent with data for the substrate specificities of neuraminidases.[21] Viral neuraminidases cleave mainly NANA $\alpha2\rightarrow3$ linked to either galactose or N-acetyl-galactosamine while bacterial neuraminidases affect $\alpha2\rightarrow3$, $\alpha2\rightarrow4$, $\alpha2\rightarrow6$ or $\alpha2\rightarrow8$ linkages of NANA to these and other sugars. Since the sialiated carbohydrates attached to most red cell membrane proteins involve $\alpha2\rightarrow3$ and $\alpha2\rightarrow6$ linkages of NANA to galactose and N-acetyl-galactosamine respectively (Fig 1), it would seem more logical for NANA-dependent glycoprotein antigens to be sensitive to either both types of neuraminidases or more sensitive to bacterial than viral neuraminidase. This would imply that the Lutheran antigens are probably not on proteins and are either dependent on NANA that is in α ketosidic linkages other than (2→3), or that the dependence is on O-acetylated neuraminic acid. Alternative linkages for NANA are more often found on the sialiated complex carbohydrates found in glycolipids, and Marcus et al[41] have reported finding Lu^b antigen activity in red cell gangliosides (Fig 2), most of which contain the lactoneotetraosyl structure (ie, paragloboside, sialosyl-paragloboside and more complex glycosphingolipids).

Chido and Rodgers antigens on red cells have been found to be sensitive to most proteolytic enzymes (Table 6). The location of these antigens on the portion of the α4 chain of the C4 component of complement[108] sensitive to trypsin treatment complies with the serologic data.

The A, B, H, I and i antigens have been found to be resistant to neuraminidase and proteolytic enzymes. The biochemistry of these antigens has been defined on red cells by using exoglycosidases other than neuraminidase, and the endoglycosidase endo-β-galactosidase (Table 2). The blood group activity of these antigens reside in terminal trisaccharides[109] or tetrasaccharides[110] in complex oligosaccharides on glycoproteins and glycolipids (Fig 2). The exoenzymes (eg, α-L-fucosidase) remove the specific terminal immunodominant carbohydrate responsible for the ABH antigen activities and uncover the carbohydrate chains which define the I antigen complex.[39] Endo-β-galactosidase cleaves larger portions of these carbohydrate chains and results in the destruction of A, B, H and I antigens. It was through the use of this enzyme that the association of I to i antigens was determined. I and i oligosaccharide chains are identical in carbohydrate content; i is unbranched while I is a branched structure.

Using intact red cells, the Rh antigens are neuraminidase and proteolytic enzyme resistant (Table 6). However, Hughes-Jones et al[91] have demonstrated inactivation of Rh antigens by treatment of red cell stroma with phospholipases. This would indicate that the serologic reactivity of these antigens are phospholipid dependent. Green[111] had previously shown the dependence of Rh antigen activity on membrane lipids by demonstrating that extraction of the lipids with butanol inactivated the antigens, while subsequent addition of phospholipids resulted in regeneration of the reactivity. Plapp et al[112] have reported the association of Rh antigens with a low molecular weight protein that comigrates with the lipid zone on SDS-PAGE while Victoria et al[113] found Rh antigen associated with band 3 glycoprotein of human red cell membrane. The protein nature of Rh antigens has been established but exact biochemistry and sterochemistry has not yet been resolved.

The other antigens listed in Table 6 that have fairly consistently been found to be denatured by proteolytic enzymes are Yt^a, JMH and Xg^a. No work has been reported on the biochemistry of these antigens.

Enhancement of Red Cell Antigen-Antibody Reactions

The most common methods for observing red cell antigen-antibody reactions consist of detecting in vitro hemolysis, direct hemagglutination or indirect hemagglutination. Enzyme treatment of red cells can cause enhancement of all of these antibody detection systems.

Antibody-mediated in vitro hemolysis is caused by activation of the classical complement pathway by binding of IgM, IgG1 or IgG3 antibodies to the red cell membrane.[114] Most anti-Tj^a (PP_1 P^k) antibodies and some anti-Vel, anti-A and anti-A,B antibodies can cause in vitro hemolysis of untreated incompatible red cells. Some anti-A, anti-A,B, anti-Lewis and anti-Kidd antibodies will only hemolyse enzyme-treated incompatible red cells. It is unclear why some red cell bound antibodies of IgM, IgG_1 or IgG_3 classes cause the activation of complement while others do not, and equally unclear why some of the complement activating antibodies will cause in vitro hemolysis while others do not. However, presumably, the more antibody that is bound to the red cell membrane, the more complement can be activated and the greater the chance that hemolysis will occur. Increased amounts of antibody binding to enzyme modified antigen positive red cells has been reported with anti-I, anti-i and anti-D antibodies,[32-35] and probably occurs with many of the blood group antibodies whose corresponding antigens are not denatured by enzymes. Another potential contributing factor for enhanced in vitro hemolysis may be the slightly increased fragility of enzyme-treated red cells.[25]

Hemagglutination is the classic method of testing for red cell antigen-antibody reactions. Stable hemagglutination will occur when multiple antibody bridges are formed between red cells and this binding force is greater than the forces driving red cells apart.[115-116] The agglutination reaction occurs in two stages: (1) sensitization or binding of antibody molecules to the antigenic determinant on the red cell membrane; (2) agglutination or crosslinking of red cells by many antibody molecules attaching by at least one combining site onto one red cell and another combining site onto another red cell (Fig 4). IgM antibody molecules are relatively large (350Å), flexible, have ten antigen combining sites, and are often capable of causing "direct" agglutination of saline suspended red cells by spanning the intercellular distances found under those conditions. In contrast, IgG antibody molecules are smaller (250Å), less flexible, have only two antigen com-

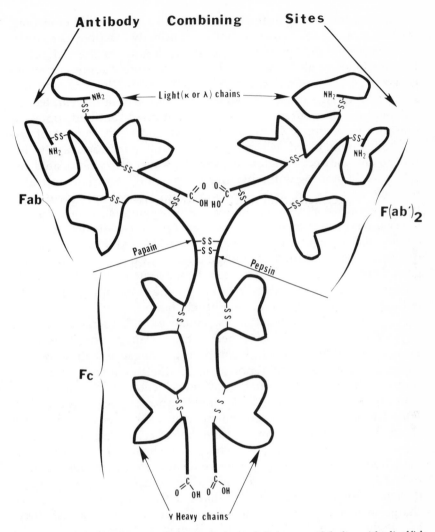

Antibody Combining Sites

Light(κ or λ) chains

Fab

F(ab')₂

Papain

Pepsin

Fc

γ Heavy chains

Fig 4.—Diagrammatic representation of human IgG immunoglobulin with disulfide bonds and enzyme cleavage sites.[117-118]

bining sites, and only infrequently cause direct agglutination of saline suspended red cells. IgG "sensitizing" antibodies are detected by an "indirect" agglutination method. Crosslinking of the sensitized red cells is brought about by an antibody (antihuman globulin serum) directed against the immunoglobulin attached to the red cells (indirect antiglobulin test).

Enzyme treatment of red cells has been found to enhance both direct[3] and indirect agglutination of red cells.[45] One effect of enzyme treatment of red cells on some antigen-antibody reactions is to cause an increase in the quantity of antibody bound to the red cells.[33] Hughes-Jones et al[120] interpret this data to simply represent an increase in association rate and equilibrium constant due to a reduction in steric hindrance caused by enzymatic removal of carbohydrates and polypeptides. Masouredis[34] suggests that increased antibody uptake is due to uncovering of latent antigens. An increased amount of IgG antibody bound to red cells can therefore result in increased agglutination in the indirect antiglobulin test. However, enzyme-treated red cells are also more agglutinable in the antiglobulin test than untreated red cells even if comparable levels of antibody and antiglobulin are bound to each.[121] Similarly, although direct agglutination of untreated red cells has been shown to be dependent on antigen site density,[115,122] enhanced direct agglutination of enzyme-treated red cells is not simply due to increased antibody binding because of exposure of latent antigens. Direct agglutination has been demonstrated with IgG antibody sensitized enzyme treated red cells but not the same untreated red cells with up to 10 to 15 times more antibody bound.[34,120,123-124]

A more popular explanation for enhanced direct agglutination of enzyme treated red cells is related to the distance normally existing between red cells. In a saline solution, the distance maintained between red cells has been reported to be due to either the repulsive forces of the electrostatic charges at red cell surfaces,[125] or the vicinal water (water of hydration) at the highly polar surface of red cells.[116] Pollack et al[125] propose that enzymatic removal of NANA, the principal charged membrane component, from the red cell membrane results in a reduction of the net negative charge which can be measured by a reduction in zeta potential. The reduction in charge results in a reduced intercellular distance and IgG molecules can now span this distance. Other investigators[126-128] have demonstrated that cell surface charge cannot be the only mechanism involved in enhanced direct hemagglutination. They found that neuraminidase-treated red cells had a lower net negative charge than protease-treated red cells, yet protease-treated red cells demonstrated greater direct agglutination than the same cells treated with neuraminidase. This could be a function of the amount of material cleaved from the cell membrane. Proteolytic enzymes remove polypeptide stems plus all NANA that was attached to the stems. Neuraminidase removes NANA but leaves the polypeptide stems. These stems might cause steric hindrance, either to the antigen-antibody reaction[126] or to the agglutination reaction.[127] The vicinal water proponents believe that enzymatic removal of

NANA and SGPs causes a reduction of vicinal water with a resultant decrease in intercellular distances. Proteolytic enzymes cause greater enhancement of direct agglutination than neuraminidase because the release of more polar material by the proteolytic enzymes results in a greater reduction in vicinal water.

Other factors besides just immunoglobulin size and intercellular distances may affect the complex physiochemical reaction of hemagglutination. Multiple antibody bridges are required for stable agglutination to occur.[115] Factors that could affect the formation of multiple bridging include cell surface shape, deformability and antigen site clustering. Van Oss and Mohn[26] have demonstrated cell surface shape changes in papain-treated red cells and propose that these changes can result in establishment of intercellular contact, which they feel is the first step in hemagglutination.[129] Other investigators[130] have demonstrated large areas of contact between enzyme treated red cells (papain-treated red cells have larger areas of contact than neuraminidase-treated cells) and this was interpreted to be due to increased membrane deformability.[31] Large areas of surface contact would facilitate the formation of multiple antibody bridges and enhance agglutination. The necessity for membrane deformability preceding hemagglutination is supported by data demonstrating that aldehyde-fixed red cells are not agglutinated by saline-agglutinating antibodies or in the indirect antiglobulin test.[116] Another factor that could affect stable agglutination is antigen site clustering. If antigen sites were found in clusters or were able to cluster after antibody attachment, multiple antibody bridging in a localized area would occur and could contribute to stronger bonding. D antigen clustering after reaction with anti-D on both red cell ghosts and intact red cells has been described.[130-132] Increased antigen clustering on enzyme-treated red cells has also been reported.[130-131] However, data from other investigators indicate that antigen clustering does not occur in intact adult red cells.[133]

An entirely different explanation for enhanced direct agglutination of enzyme-treated IgG-sensitized red cells has been proposed.[134-135] Enzyme treatment of red cells exposes membrane bound Fc receptors which can crosslink with the Fc region of the IgG immunoglobulin coating the red cells. If this were the only mechanism involved, many IgG-coated red cells should demonstrate enhanced direct agglutination using enzyme-treated red cells (if the antigens are not denatured by enzymes). However, many blood group system antibodies show no such enhancement.[94, 119]

Enhancement of direct agglutination can be demonstrated with IgM antibodies as well as IgG antibodies. The observation of IgM Rh antibodies at 37 C only with enzyme-treated red cells is fairly common.[119] Many IgM cold autoagglutinins demonstrate enhanced agglutination not only at low temperature (4-18 C) using enzyme-treated red cells, but may also demonstrate enhanced agglutination at higher temperatures (22 C or above).[33] This elevation in thermal amplitude is probably related to both increased sensitization and enhanced direct agglutination seen with enzyme-treated red cells.

"Enzyme-autoagglutinins" have been found in adult sera.[44,136-137] These antibodies are enzyme specific and react with all red cells, including the autologous red cells, that have been treated with the specific enzyme. These antibodies are not reacting with enzyme bound irreversibly to the red cell membrane, but are probably reacting with an enzyme exposed receptor that is glycoprotein.[136] If this is the case, the antigens might be more appropriately termed enzyme-cryptantigens.

A summary of antigen-antibody reaction enhancement due to enzyme modification is found in Table 9.

Table 9.—Enzyme-Induced Enhancement of Antibody Reactivity

Antibodies	Enhancement	References
ABH, P	Agglutination, thermal amplitude, hemolysis	6,44,68,119
Lewis, Kidd	Hemolysis, sensitization	44,68,119
Cold autoagglutinins	Agglutination, thermal amplitude	33,44,119
Rh auto and alloantibodies	Agglutination, sensitization	31,45-46,68,119
Enzyme autoagglutinins	Agglutination, rarely sensitization	44,136-137

Antigen "Construction" by Transferases

The biochemistry of many red cell antigens has been elucidated by the use of glycosyltransferase enzymes to construct antigens. Table 10 gives a list of transferases that have been used to study the complex ABH and Ii oligosaccharides (Fig 2), and M,N tetrasaccharides (Fig 1). Review of these studies can be found elsewhere.[140]

White Cells and Platelets

Enzymes have been useful in defining the biochemical structure of the histocompatibility antigens on white cells and glycoproteins on the

Table 10.—Glycosyltransferases Used in Immunohematology

Enzyme	Substrates	Antigen Studies
α-L-fucosyltransferase	Fucose from GDP L-fucose to carbon-2 position of β-galactosyl residue of Type 1 or 2 chain	H[11]
α-N-acetylgalactosaminyl-transferase	N-acetylgalactosamine from UDP N-acetylgalactosamine to β-galactosyl unit in H-active substance	A[11]
α-galactosyltransferase	Galactose from UDP galactose to β-galactosyl unit in H-active structure	B[11]
α-L-fucosyltransferase	Fucose from GDP fucose to carbon-4 position of N-acetylglucosamine of Type I chains	Le[a 11]
N-acetyl-D-galactosamine-β-D-galactosyltransferase	D-galactose from UDP galactose to carbon-3 position of nonreducing N-acetyl-D-galactosamine α-linked	Tn[138]
β-galactoside α2→3 sialyltransferase	NANA from CMP-NANA to α2→3 linkage with β-galactose in alkali labile tetrasaccharides	M,N[139]
α-N-acetylgalactosaminide α2→6 sialyltransferase	NANA from CMP-NANA to α2→6 linkage with α-N-acetylgalactosamine in alkali labile tetraccharides	M,N[139]

Legend: GDP = guanosine diphosphate
UDP = uridine diphosphate
CMP-NANA = cytidine-5'-monophospho-N-acetylneuraminate

platelet surface. HLA-A and -B antigens are biochemically similar to immunoglobulins and the extracellular portions of these antigens have papain cleavage sites.[141] HLA DRw antigens have been found to be glycoproteins which also have an external papain cleavage site. Glycopeptide fragments have been isolated after treating platelets with trypsin, pronase, papain, plasmin, thrombin and chymotrypsin.[142] Reviews on the biochemistry of these structures can be found elsewhere.[141-142]

Immunoglobulins

A model of a human IgG immunoglobulin molecule is given in Fig 4.[117,118] Papain, pepsin, and trypsin proteolytic enzymes have been used to identify the biochemical sequence of the proteins and the biological functions of the regions of the molecules. The IgG immunoglobulin can be divided into a number of different fragments by papain and pepsin. Papain hydrolyses the immunoglobulin into two Fab fragments and one Fc fragment. The antibody combining sites on the Fab fragments can still combine with the appropriate antigens. Pepsin treatment of the immunoglobulin occurs past an inter-heavy chain disulfide linkage resulting in the formation of one F(ab')$_2$. The Fc fragment is extensively degraded. The F(ab')$_2$ fragment is capable of combining with the appropriate antigens. A comprehensive review of the immunoglobulin structures can be found elsewhere.[117]

Applications of Enzymes

Most immunohematologists use proteolytic enzymes to treat red cells for antibody detection or identification purposes. We look for increased agglutination or sensitization with certain blood group system antibodies (Table 9) or a decrease in reactivity with others (Table 6). A review of the methods, controls and pitfalls is found elsewhere.[100]

New applications of enzymes in immunohematology have developed in the last few years. Some of these involve new or practical applications of old methods while others are the application of methods not commonly used in immunohematology.

Two practical applications of enzyme methods involving the ABH blood group system have recently been reported. Valko et al[143] have reported a simple procedure for detection of B- gene specified transferases in serum of individuals whose genetic ABH group may not be easily detectable from red cell agglutination studies (ie, subgroups, chimeras, O$_h$ individuals). They demonstrated the presence of α-galactosyltransferase in serum by converting group O red cells to B-active cells upon incubation of the serum-cell mixture with UDP D-galactose (Table 10). Conversely, the action of α-galactosidase found in green coffee beans (Table 2) has been applied to the practical problems of blood transfusion. Group B red cells were converted to group O red cells by this exoglycosidase and were found to survive normally in A, B, and O individuals.[144]

Another new application of enzymes is removal of IgG molecules from red cells.[106] Papain treatment of sensitized red cells cleaves the Fc fragment, the fragment that normally reacts with anti-IgG antihuman globulin serum, but does not result in the dissociation of the resultant Fab fragments (Fig 4). With the knowledge that interchain disulfide bonds can be split by sulfhydryl compounds,[145] Branch and Petz mixed high concentrations of a sulfhydryl reagent with papain (ZZAP) and

162

treated IgG-sensitized red cells. This method reduced the strength of the direct antiglobulin test more effectively than by treating the sensitized red cells with equivalent concentrations of either the enzyme or sulfhydryl compound alone. This could be a result of disruption of the inter-light and heavy chain disulfide bonds which could then cause dissociation of the Fab combining sites (Fig 4). Another possibility is that intrachain disulfide bonds in the light chains and heavy chains are disrupted allowing further proteolytic digestion of the Fab fragment which ultimately results in dissociation.

Recently, a new procedure using enzymes has been applied to the detection of antigen-antibody reactions. Enzyme-linked immunosorbent assay (ELISA) is based on the fact that either antigen or antibody can be linked to an enzyme, and the resultant complex retains both immunological and enzymatic activity. Antigen and antibody are allowed to react and excess reactants are removed. A substrate is added that develops a color change upon digestion by the enzyme, and the optical density of the product can then be measured.[146] This methodology has been applied to detection of hepatitis B surface antigen[147] and as an indirect method for detecting IgG-immunoglobulin-coating red cels.[148] The enzyme-linked antiglobulin test (ELAT) has recently been applied to quantitation of antibodies on red cells and platelets,[149-151] comparison of antibody elution techniques,[152] and detection of mixed red cell populations.[153] This new methodology is objective and can be automated, but is more time-consuming than the standard antiglobulin technique.

Another unusual application of an enzyme test has recently been reported. Marsh et al[154] have reported an association between the X-linked McLeod red cell phenotype and increased levels of serum creatine phosphokinase (CPK) isoenzyme type MM. Eleven males with McLeod syndrome had from 3 to 13 times greater CPK levels than the upper limit of normal, and Marsh concludes that this is associated with a muscle cell anomaly. This serum enzyme test, associated with the acanthocytic morphology of the red cells, could be used in the laboratory as screening tests for McLeod syndrome.

Conclusion

We have unknowingly used enzymes to assist us since ancient Greek times. For many years we have used enzymes in immunohematology because of the serological effects obtained using enzyme-treated red cells, without understanding why antigens were denatured or reactivity was enhanced. Recently, we have begun to understand enzymatic mechanisms and have been applying them to the elucidation of the biochemistry of blood components. Many of the problems associated with the progress in these areas have been related to isolation and purification of the reactants, since both the enzymes and the substrates may only be present in small quantities. The new hybridoma methodology for producing unlimited quantities of monospecific antibodies,[155] the technology for linking these antibodies to columns (affinity chromotography),[5] and the technology for solubilizing membranes without destroying the antigenic portions of the cell surfaces,[42] will allow us to continue to isolate and purify these proteins and carbohydrates. Enzymes will continue to be used to assist in these exciting biochemical investigations.

Acknowledgments

I would like to thank W.D. Dean, J.L. Fletcher, J. La Rochelle, J. Miller, M. Reid and E. Sugasawara for their suggestions during preparation of this manuscript, and M. Rees-White for typing of this manuscript.

References

1. Koshland DE, Jr. Enzymes. In: The new encyclopedia britannica macropaedia. Chicago: Helen Hemingway Benton, 1974;6:896-902.
2. Perham RN. The protein chemistry of enzymes. FEBS Lett 1976; 62:E20-9.
3. Pickles MM. Effect of cholera filtrate on red cells as demonstrated by incomplete Rh antibodies. Nature 1946;158:880.
4. Porter RR. The formation of a specific inhibitor by hydrolysis of rabbit antiovalbumin. Biochem J 1950;46:479-84.
5. Stryer L. Biochemistry. San Francisco: Freeman, 1981.
6. Lewis AJ. Papain, ficin and bromelain in the detection of incomplete Rhesus antibodies. Br J Haematol 1957;3:332-9.
7. Nomenclature Committee of the International Union of Biochemistry. 1978 enzyme nomenclature recommendations. New York: Academic Press, 1979.
8. Sigma Chemical Company. Biochemical and organic compounds for research and diagnostic clinical reagents. 1982.

9. Miles Laboratories, Inc. Biochemicals Immunochemicals. 1981.

10. Springer GF, Ansell NJ. Inactivation of human erythrocyte agglutinogens M and N by influenza viruses and receptor destroying enzyme. Proc Natl Acad Sci USA 1958;44:182-9.

11. Watkins WM. Blood group substances: their nature and genetics. In: Surgenor DM, ed. The red blood cell. 2nd ed. New York: Academic Press, 1974;1:293-360.

12. Watanabe K, Hakomori S, Childs RA, et al. Characterization of a blood group I-active ganglioside: structural requirements for I and i specificities. J Biol Chem 1979;254:3221-8.

13. Andreu G, Doinel C, Cartron JP, et al. Induction of T_k polyagglutination by Bacteroides fragilis culture supernatants: associated modifications of ABH and Ii antigens. Rev Fr Transfus Immunohematol 1979;23:551-61.

14. Fukuda MN, Fukada M, Hakomori S. Cell surface modification by endo-β-galactosidase. Change of blood group activities and release of oligosaccharides from glycoproteins and sphingoglycolipids of human erythrocytes. J Biol Chem 1979;254:5458-65.

15. Keil B. Proteolysis—one of the major tools of physiological regulation. In: Agarwal MK, ed. Proteases and hormones. Amsterdam: Elsevier/North-Holland Biomedical Press, 1979:1-17.

16. Glazer AN, Smith EL. Papain and other plant sulfhydryl proteolytic enzymes. In: Boyer PD, ed. The enzymes. 3rd ed. New York: Academic Press, 1970;3:502-46.

17. Hughes & Hughes (Enzymes) Ltd. Stem Bromelain; Bromelase. 12a High Street, Brentwood, Essex.

18. Dreuth J, Jansonius JN, Koeboek R, et al. Papain, x-ray structure. In: Boyer PD, ed. The enzymes. 3rd ed. New York: Academic Press, 1970;3:484-501.

19. Morton JA, Pickles MM. Use of trypsin in the detection of incomplete anti-Rh antibodies. Nature 1947;159:779-80.

20. Judson PA, Anstee DJ. Comparative effect of trypsin and chymotrypsin on blood group antigens. Med Lab Sci 1977;34:1-6.

21. Drzeniek R. Substrate specificity of neuraminidases. Histochem J 1973;5:271-90.

22. Markland FS Jr, Smith EL. Subtilisins: primary structure, chemical and physical properties. In: Boyer PD, ed. The enzymes. 3rd ed. New York; Academic Press, 1970;3:562-608.

23. Steane SM. Basic membrane biochemistry and its relationship to blood group serology. In: Bell CA, ed. A seminar on antigens on blood cells and body fluids. Washington, DC: American Association of Blood Banks, 1980:1-24.

24. Makinodan T, Macris NT. The effect of ficin on the agglutination of human red blood cells. J Immunol 1955;75:192-6.
25. Ponder E. Effects produced by trypsin on certain properties of the human red cell. Blood 1951;6:350-6.
26. van Oss CJ, Mohn JF. Scanning electron microscopy of red cell agglutination. Vox Sang 1970;19:432-43.
27. Cook GMW, Heard DH, Seaman GVF. Sialic acids and the electrokinetic charge of the human erythrocyte. Nature 1961;191:44-7.
28. Mäkelä O, Miettinen T, Pesola R. Release of sialic acid and carbohydrates from human red cells by trypsin treatment. Vox Sang 1960;5:492-6.
29. Springer GF. Enzymatic and nonenzymatic alterations of erythrocyte surface antigens. Bacteriol Rev 1963;27:191-227.
30. Doinel C, Andreu G, Cartron JP, et al. T_k polyagglutination produced in vitro by an endo-beta-galactosidase. Vox Sang 1980; 38:94-8.
31. Masouredis SP, Sudora EJ, Victoria EJ. Immunological and electron microscopic analysis of IgG anti-D saline hemagglutination of neuraminidase—and protease—modified red cells. J Lab Clin Med 1977;90:929-48.
32. Doinel C, Ropars C, Salmon CH. Effects of proteolytic enzymes and neuraminidase on I and i erythrocyte antigen sites. Quantitative and thermodynamic studies. Immunology 1978;34:653-62.
33. Wheeler WE, Luhby AL, Scholl MLL. The action of enzymes in hemagglutinating systems: II. agglutinating properties of trypsin-modified red cells with anti-Rh sera. J Immunol 1958;65: 39-46.
34. Masouredis SP. Reaction of I^{131} anti-Rh_0(D) with enzyme treated red cells. Transfusion 1962;2:363-74.
35. Coffin SF, Pickles MM. The ability of trypsin to restore specific agglutinating capacity of erythrocytes treated with periodate. J Immunol 1953;71:177-82.
36. Anstee DJ. The blood group MNSs-active sialoglycoproteins. Semin Hematol 1981;18:13-31.
37. Thomas DB, Winzler RJ. Structural studies on human erythrocyte glycoproteins. J Biol Chem 1969;244:5943-6.
38. Dahr W, Beyreuther K, Steinbach H, et al. Structure of the Ss blood group antigens: II. A methionine/threonine polymorphism within the N-terminal sequence of the Ss glycoprotein. Hoppe Seylers Z Physiol Chem 1980;361:895-906.
39. Hakomori S. Blood group ABH and Ii antigens of human eryth-

rocytes: chemistry, polymorphism, and their developmental change. Semin Hematol 1981;18:39-62.

40. Marcus DM, Naiki M, Kundu SK. Abnormalities in the glyco-sphingolipid content of human P^k and p erythrocytes. Proc Natl Acad Sci USA 1976;73:3263-7.

41. Marcus DM, Kundu SK, Suzuki A. The P blood group system: recent progress in immunochemistry and genetics. Semin Hematol 1981;18:63-71.

42. Rolih SD. Erythrocyte antigens of the MN system and related structures. In: Bell CA, ed. A seminar on antigens on blood cells and body fluids. Washington, DC: American Association of Blood Banks, 1980:209-47.

43. Springer GF, Stalder K. Action of influenza viruses, receptor de-stroying enzyme and proteases on blood group agglutinogen Mg. Nature 1961;191:187-8.

44. Rosenfield RE, Vogel P. The identification of hemagglutinins with red cells altered with trypsin. Trans NY Acad Sci 1951;13: 213-20.

45. Unger MD, Katz L. The effect of trypsin on hemagglutinogens determining eight blood group systems. J Lab Clin Med 1952; 39:135-41.

46. Morton JA, Pickles MM. The proteolytic enzyme test for detecting incomplete antibodies. J Clin Pathol 1951;4:189-99.

47. Evans RS, Turner E, Bingham M. Studies with radioiodinated cold agglutinins of ten patients. Am J Med 1965;38:378-95.

48. Roelcke D, Uhlenbruck G. Proteinase K: a new serologically effec-tive protease from fungi. Z Med Mikrobiol Immunol 1960;155: 156-70. (German)

49. Marcus DM, Kabat EA, Rosenfield RE. The action of enzymes from Clostridium tertium on the I antigenic determinant of human erythrocytes. J Exp Med 1963;118:175-9.

50. Roelcke D. The Lud cold agglutinin: a further antibody recogniz-ing N-acetylneuraminic acid-determined antigens not fully ex-pressed at birth. Vox Sang 1981;41:316-8.

51. Marsh WL, Jenkins WJ. Anti-Sp$_1$: the recognition of a new cold autoantibody. Vox Sang 1968;15:177-86.

52. Roelcke D. Pr and Gd antigens. Bld Transf Immunohaematol 1981;24:27-36.

53. Habibi B, Cregut R, Brossard Y, et al. Auto-anti-Pr$_a$: a 'second' example in a newborn. Br J Haematol 1975;30:499-505.

54. Badakere SS, Parab BB, Bhatia HM. Further observations on the In^a(Indian) antigen in populations. Vox Sang 1974;26:400-3.

55. Bhatia HM, Badakere SS, Mokoshi SA, et al. Studies on the blood group antigen In[a]. Immunol Commun 1980;9:203-15.
56. Giles CM. Antithetical relationship of anti-In[a] with the Salis antibody. Vox Sang 1975;29:73-6.
57. Issitt PD, Issitt CH, Moulds J, et al. Some observations on the T, Tn and Sd[a] antigens and the antibodies that define them. Transfusion 1972;12:217-21.
58. Judd WJ, McGuire-Mallory D, Anderson KM, et al. Concomitant T- and Tk-activation associated with acquired-B antigens. Transfusion 1979;19:293-8.
59. Myllyla G, Furuhjelm U, Nordling S, et al. Persistent mixed field polyagglutinability: electrokinetic and serological aspects. Vox Sang 1971;20:7-23.
60. Sturgeon P, McQuiston DT, Taswell HF, et al. Permanent mixed-field polyagglutinability (PMFP) I. Serological observations. Vox Sang 1973;25:481-497.
61. Issitt PD, Pavone BG, Wagstaff W, et al. The phenotypes En(a−), Wr(a−b−), and En(a+), Wr(a+b−), and further studies on the Wright and En blood group systems. Transfusion 1976;16:396-407.
62. Issitt PD. The MN Blood Group System. Cincinnati: Montgomery Scientific Publications, 1981.
63. Vyas GN, Fudenberg HH. Use of B subtilis neutral proteinase in blood group serology. Vox Sang 1968;15:300-3.
64. Strohm PL, Busch S. Comparison of effectiveness of various proteolytic enzymes in blood-group antibody detection. Transfusion 1969;9:93-7.
65. Hirsch W, Moores P, Sanger R, et al. Notes on some reactions of human anti-M and anti-N sera. Br J Haematol 1957;3:134-42.
66. Dahr W, Uhlenbruck G, Wagstaff W, et al. Studies on the membrane glycoprotein defect on En(a−) erythrocytes: II. MN antigenic properties of En(a−) erythrocytes. J Immunogenet 1976;3:383-93.
67. Issitt PD, Jerez GC. Absorption of unwanted antibodies from sera containing MNS or Duffy group antibodies without need for selecting "appropriately negative" cells. Transfusion 1966;6:155-9.
68. Morton JA. Some observations on the action of blood group antibodies on red cells treated with proteolytic enzymes. Br J Haematol 1962;8:134-48.
69. Giles CM, Howell P. An antibody in the serum of an MN patient which reacts with the M_1 antigen. Vox Sang 1974;27:43-51.

70. Dahr W, Uhlenbruck G, Knott H. Immunochemical aspects of the MNSs-blood group system. J Immunogenet 1975;2:87-100.
71. Prager MD, Soules ML, Fletcher MA. Further studies on the mechanism of the effect of enzymes on erythrocyte serology with special reference to pronase. Transfusion 1968;8:220-5.
72. Anstee DJ. Blood group MNSs-active sialoglycoproteins of the human erythrocyte membrane. In: Sandler SG, Nusbacher J, Schanfield MS, eds. Immunobiology of the erythrocyte. New York: AR Liss, 1980:67-98.
73. Wallace J, Izatt MM. The Cl^a (Caldwell) antigen: a new rare human blood group antigen related to the MNSs system. Nature 1963;200:689-90.
74. Skov F. A new rare blood group antigen, Je^a. Vox Sang 1972;23: 461-3.
75. Orjasaeter H, Kornstad L, Heier AM. Studies on the Ny^a blood group antigen and antibodies. Vox Sang 1964;9:673-83.
76. Dybkjaer E, Poole J, Giles CM. A new Miltenberger class detected by a second example of Anek type serum. Vox Sang 1981;41: 302-5.
77. Bowley CC, Griffith RW. A case of haemolytic disease of the newborn due to anti-Verweyst. Vox Sang 1962;7:373-4.
78. Chattoraj A, Kamat M, Summaria L, et al. Studies on the agglutination of erythrocytes treated with human plasmin and some other enzymes. Proc Soc Exp Biol Med 1969;130:1315-8.
79. Colledge KI, Pezzulich M, Marsh WL. Anti-Fy^5, an antibody disclosing a probable association between the Rhesus and Duffy blood group genes. Vox Sang 1973;24:193-9.
80. Mann JD, Cahan A, Gelb AG, et al. A sex-linked blood group. Lancet 1962;i:8-10.
81. Habibi B, Tippett P, Libesnerais M, et al. Protease inactivation of red cell Xg^a receptor. Abstract 15th Congress of the International Society of Blood Transfusion. Paris, 1978;2:711.
82. Middleton J, Crookston MC. Chido-substance in plasma. Vox Sang 1972;23:256-61.
83. Moulds MK. Special serological technics useful in resolving high-titer, low-avidity antibodies. In: High-titer, low-avidity antibodies: recognition and resolution. Washington, DC: American Association of Blood Banks, 1979:33-43.
84. Longster G, Giles CM. A new specificity; anti-Rg^a, reacting with a red cell and serum antigen. Vox Sang 1976;30:175-80.
85. Giles CM, Metaxas-Bühler, Romanski Y, et al. Studies on the Yt blood group system. Vox Sang 1967;13:171-80.

86. Eaton BR, Morton JA, Pickles MM, et al. A new antibody, anti-Yt^a, characterizing a blood-group antigen of high incidence. Br J Haematol 1956;2:333-41.

87. Sabo B, Moulds JJ, McCreary J. Anti-JMH: another high titer-low avidity antibody against a high frequency antigen. Transfusion 1978;18:387.

88. Molthan L, Giles CM. A new antigen, Yk^a (York), and its relationship to Cs^a (Cost). Vox Sang 1975;29:145-53.

89. Molthan L. Anti-York (Yk^a) and other HTLA antibodies (Cs^a, McC^a, Kn^a) revisited. Transfusion 1978;18:622.

90. Boyd PA. Some serological observations of the Kidd, Rhesus and Scianna blood group systems, MS thesis. University of Cincinnati, Cincinnati, Ohio, 1980.

91. Hughes-Jones NC, Green EJ, Hunt VAM. Loss of Rh antigen activity following the action of phospholipase A$_2$ on red cell stroma. Vox Sang 1975;29:184-91.

92. Lambert R, Edwards J, Anstee DJ. A simple method for standardization of proteolytic enzymes used in blood group serology. Med Lab Sci 1978;35:233-8.

93. Draper EK. A simple spectrophotometric method for the standardization of proteases in common use in blood banking. Fenwal Laboratories: Winners of the 1981 American Association of Blood Banks Scholarship Awards, 1-28.

94. Issitt PD, Issitt CH. Applied Blood Group Serology. 2nd ed. Oxnard: Spectra Biologicals, 1975.

95. Steane EA. The physical chemistry of hemagglutination. In: A seminar on polymorphisms in human blood. Washington, DC: American Association of Blood Banks, 1975;105-27.

96. Tomita M, Marchesi VT. Amino acid sequence and oligosaccharide attachment sites of human erythrocyte glycophorin. Proc Nat Acad Sci USA 1975;72:2964-8.

97. Dahr W, Issitt PD, Uhlenbruck G. New concepts of the MNSs blood group system. In: Mohn JF, Plunkett RW, Cunningham RK, Lambert RM, eds. Human blood groups. Basel: S Karger, 1977: 197-205.

98. Furthmayr, H. Structural comparison of glycophorins and immunochemical analysis of genetic variants. Nature 1978;271:519-24.

99. Dahr W, Gielen W, Beyreuther K, et al. Structure of the Ss blood group antigens: I. Isolation of Ss-active glycopeptides and differentiation of the antigens by modification of methionine. Hoppe Seylers Z Physiol Chem 1980;361:145-52.

100. Ellisor SS. Enzymes used in immunohematology. In: Rolih S, Albietz C, eds. Enzymes, inhibitions and adsorptions. Washington, DC: American Association of Blood Banks, 1981:1-37.

101. Dahr W, Uhlenbruck G, Gunson HH, et al. Molecular basis of Tn-polyagglutinability. Vox Sang 1975;29:36-50.

102. Jensen NJ, Furcht LT. Localization of the Duffy antigen on the red cell membrane components. Transfusion 1978;18:643.

103. Moore S, Woodrow CF, McClelland DBL. Isolation of membrane components associated with human red cell antigens Rh (D), (c), (E) and Fy^a. Nature 1982;295:529-31.

104. Furuhjelm U, Myllyla G, Nevanlinna HR, et al. The red cell phenotype En(a−) and anti-En^a: serological and physicochemical aspects. Vox Sang 1969;256-78.

105. Steck TL. The band 3 protein of the human red cell membrane: a review. Supramol Struct 1978;8:311-24.

106. Branch DR, Petz LD. A new reagent (ZZAP) having multiple applications in immunohematology. Am J Clin Pathol, (in press).

107. Advani H, Zamor J, Judd J, et al. Inactivation of Kell blood group antigens by 2-aminoethylisothiouronium bromide. Br J Haematol 1982;51:107-15.

108. Chu VFH, Marsh WL, Gigli I. Chido and Rodgers antigenic determinant of the fourth component of human complement. J Immunol 1982;128:181-5.

109. Kabat EA, Liao J, Burzynska MH, et al. Immunochemical studies on blood groups: LXIX. The conformation of the trisaccharide determinant in the combining site of anti-I Ma (group 1). Mol Immunol 1981;18:873-81.

110. Watkins WM. Genetic regulation of the structure of blood group-specific glycoproteins. Biochem Soc Symp 1974;40:125-46.

111. Green FA. Erythrocyte membrane lipids and Rh antigen activity. J Biol Chem 1972;247:881-7.

112. Plapp FV, Kowalski MM, Tilzer L, et al. Partial purification of Rh$_o$(D) antigen from Rh positive and Rh negative erythrocytes. Proc Natl Acad Sci USA 1979;76:2964-8.

113. Victoria EJ, Mahan LC, Masouredis SP. Anti-Rho(D) binds to band 3 glycoprotein of the human erythrocyte membrane. Proc Natl Acad Sci USA 1981;78:2898-902.

114. Garratty G. Erythrocyte-bound complement components in health and disease. In: Sandler SG, Nusbacher J, Schanfield MS, eds. Immunobiology of the erythrocyte. New York: AR Liss 1980: 133-55.

115. Greenbury CL, Moore DH, Nunn LAC. Reaction of 7S and 19S components of immune rabbit antisera with human group A and AB red cells. Immunology 1963;6:421-33.
116. Steane EA, Greenwalt TJ. Erythrocyte agglutination. In: Sandler SG, Nusbacher J, Schanfield MS, eds. Immunobiology of the erythrocyte. New York: AR Liss, 1980:171-88.
117. Gally JA. Structure of immunoglobulins. In: Sela M, ed. The antigens. New York: Academic Press, 1973;1:161-298.
118. Hobart MJ, McConnell I. The immune system: a course on the molecular and cellular basis of immunity. Oxford: Blackwell Scientific Publications, 1975.
119. Mollison PL. Blood transfusion in clinical medicine. 6th ed. Oxford: Blackwell Scientific Publications, 1979.
120. Hughes-Jones NC, Gardner B, Telford R. The effect of ficin on the reaction between anti-D and red cells. Vox Sang 1964;9:175-82.
121. Rearden A, Masouredis SP. The antiglobulin reaction with native and enzyme-modified red cells. Transfusion 1980;20:377-83.
122. Hoyer LN, Trabold NC. The significance of erythrocyte antigen site density. J Clin Invest 1970;49:87-95.
123. Pirofsky B, Cordova M, Imel TL. The function of proteolytic enzymes and tannic acid in inducing erythrocyte agglutination. J Immunol 1962;89:767-74.
124. Masouredis SP. Red cell membrane blood group antigens. In: Membrane structure and function of human blood cells. Washington, DC: American Association of Blood Banks, 1976:37-60.
125. Pollack W, Hager HJ, Reckel R, et al. A study of the forces involved in the second stage of hemagglutination. Transfusion 1965;5:158-83.
126. Stratton F, Rawlinson VI, Gunson HH, et al. The role of zeta potential in Rh agglutination. Vox Sang 1973;24:273-9.
127. Luner SJ, Sturgeon P, Szrlarek D, et al. Effects of proteases and neuraminidase on RBC surface charge and agglutination: A kinetic study. Vox Sang 1975;28:184-99.
128. Steane EA, Greenwalt TJ. Red cell agglutination. In: Mohn JF, Plunkett RW, Cunningham RK, Lambert RM, eds. Human blood groups. Basel: S Karger, 1977:36-43.
129. van Oss CJ, Mohn JF, Cunningham RK. Influence of various physiochemical factors on hemagglutination. Vox Sang 1978;34:351-61.
130. Voak D, Cawley JC, Emmines JP, et al. The role of enzymes and albumin in haemagglutination reactions. Vox Sang 1974;27:156-70.

131. Victoria EJ, Muchmore EA, Sudora EJ, et al. The role of antigen mobility in anti-Rh$_0$(D)-induced agglutination. J Clin Invest 1975;56:292-301.

132. Makler MT, Pesce AJ. Scanning electron microscopy shows that both antigen mobility and membrane deformation occur in hemagglutination reaction. Vox Sang 1981;40:1-5.

133. Schekman R, Singer SJ. Clustering and endocytosis of membrane receptors can be induced in mature erythrocytes of neonatal but not adult humans. Proc Natl Acad Sci USA 1976;73:4075-9.

134. Wiener AS, Katz L. Studies on the use of enzyme-treated red cells in tests for Rh sensitization. J Immunol 1951;66:51-66.

135. Margni RA, Leoni J, Bazzurro M. The incomplete anti-Rh antibody agglutination mechanism of trypsinized O Rh+ red cells. Immunology 1977;33:153-60.

136. Mellbye OJ. Properties of the trypsinized red cell receptor reacting in reversible agglutination by normal sera. Scand J Haematol 1969;6:139-48.

137. Mellbye OJ. Specificity of natural agglutinins against red cells modified by trypsin and other agents. Scand J Haematol 1969; 6:166-72.

138. Cartron JP, Andreu G, Cartron J, et al. Demonstration of T-transferase deficiency in Tn-polyagglutinable blood samples. Eur J Biochem 1978;92:111-9.

139. Sadler JE, Paulson JC, Hill RL. The role of sialic acid in the expression of human MN blood group antigens. J Biol Chem 1979;254:2112-9.

140. Beyer TA, Sandler JE, Rearick JI, et al. Glycosyltransferases and their use in assessing oligsaccharide structure and structure-function relationships. In: Meister A, ed. Advances in enzymology and related areas of molecular biology. New York: John Wiley and Sons, 1981:23-175.

141. Owen MJ, Crumpton MJ. Biochemistry of major human histocompatibility antigens. Immunol Today 1980;1:117-22.

142. Jamieson GA. The platelet. In: Jamieson GA, Robinson DM, eds. Mammalian cell membranes: surface membranes of specific cell types. London: Butterworths, 1977:27-46.

143. Valko DA, Rolih SD, Moulds JJ, et al. A simple method for detection of the B-gene specified transferase enzyme. Transfusion 1981;21:624.

144. Goldstein J, Siviglia G, Hurst R, et al. Group B erythrocytes enzymatically converted to group O survive normally in A, B and O individuals. Science 1982;215:168-70.

145. Nisonoff A, Wissler FC, Woernley DL. Mechanism of formation of univalent fragments of rabbit antibody. Biochem Biophy Res Commun 1959;1:318-22.

146. Engvall E, Pesce AJ, eds. Quantitative enzyme immunoassay. Oxford: Blackwood Scientific Publication, 1978. From Scand J Immunol 1978;8(supp 7).

147. Walters G, Kuijers L, Kacaki J, et al. Solid-phase enzyme-immunoassay for detection of hepatitis B surface antigen. J Clin Pathol 1976;29:873-9.

148. Leikola J, Perkins HA. Enzyme-linked antiglobulin test: an accurate and simple method to quantify red cell antibodies. Transfusion 1980;20:138-44.

149. Nason S, Chen S, Peetoom F. A solid-phase enzyme immunoassay for quantitation of red blood cell and platelet associated IgG. Transfusion 1981;21:599-60.

150. Crow CA, Perkins HA, Leikola J. A sensitive enzyme immunoassay for the detection of red blood cell IgG sensitization. Transfusion 1981;21:626-7.

151. Brown PJ, Bodensteiner DC, Plapp FV. Enzyme-linked immunosorbent assay detection of antibody bound in vivo in patients with hemolytic anemias. Transfusion 1981;21:627.

152. Gibble JW, Salamon JL, Ness PM. Comparison of antibody elution techniques by enzyme-linked antiglobulin test (ELAT). Transfusion 1981;21:627.

153. Huang ST, Floyd DM, Poom MC. Detection of mixed red cell populations by two enzyme-linked immunochemical methods. Transfusion 1981;21:627-8.

154. Marsh WL, Marsh NJ, Moore A, et al. Elevated serum creative phosphokinase in subjects with McLeod syndrome. Vox Sang 1981;40:403-11.

155. Giusti AM, Zack DJ, Scharff MD. The production and use of monoclonal antibodies. In: Hybridomas and monoclonal antibodies. Washington, DC: American Association of Blood Banks, 1981:1-10.

8

Elution of Antibody from Red Cells

W. John Judd, FIMLS, MI Biol

Introduction

ELUTION OF ANTIBODY from sensitized red cells has wide application in immunohematology, particularly in the evaluation of blood samples with a positive direct antiglobulin test (DAT). In conjunction with an appropriate adsorption procedure, elution techniques also may be used for the purification of blood group antibodies, the detection of weakly expressed antigens, and the resolution of sera containing multiple antibody specificities. Further, since the sensitivity of a combined adsorption-elution procedure is not readily surpassed by any other routine serological test, the results obtained can be considered virtually diagnostic when such studies are used to confirm antibody specificity, or to establish that red cells are devoid of a particular blood group antigen.

Numerous methods, and minor variations thereof, have been described for the effective elution of antibody from red cells, the objective of all procedures being to dissociate red cell antigen-antibody complexes without causing significant destruction of antibody molecules. To this end, methods utilizing heat, hapten addition, freeze-thawing, organic solvents, sonication, high salt concentrations and extreme variation of pH, have been employed.

In this chapter, the technical and theoretical aspects of elution tests will be discussed, and the applications of elution in immunohematology will be reviewed.

Historical Review

Most blood bank technologists will be familiar with the heat elution technique attributed to Landsteiner and Miller.[1] This is probably the

W. John Judd, FIMLS, MI Biol, Associate Professor of Medical Technology and Director, Blood Bank Reference Laboratory, Department of Pathology, The University of Michigan Medical School, Ann Arbor, Michigan

first description of an elution technique written in English, although the paper cites a reference to its use by Landsteiner (written in German) as early as 1902.

It was not until 1947, when Kidd[2] modified the technique of Landsteiner and van der Scheer[3] for the dissociation of azostromato-antibody complexes, that an alternative method for antibody elution from red cells was reported. This technique involved freeze-thaw lysis of antibody-coated red cells, precipitation of the stroma with 1 N HCl, elution of antibody from the stroma using a citrate-HCl buffer at pH 3.2-3.4, and neutralization of the eluate with 5 N NaOH. Modifications to the elution phase of this procedure were reported by Komninos and Rosenthal,[4] who used 8% NaCl with subsequent dialysis of the eluate against normal saline to restore tonicity, and by Vos and Kelsall,[5] who eluted stromal-bound antibody with ether. In addition, the literature contains references to procedures by van Loghem et al[6] and Selwyn,[7] which are not well documented, but appear to be based on Kidd's method[2] for the preparation of red cell stroma. All of these methods are reported to produce virtually hemoglobin-free eluates.

Obtaining hemoglobin-free eluates from antibody-coated red cells to permit immunochemical as well as serological analysis of the eluted material also appears to have been the objective of a number of other investigators. Greenwalt[8] used a mixture of distilled water and toluene to precipitate stroma, harvested the precipitate by filtration on glass wool, and recovered bound antibody into either saline or 8% albumin by elution at 56 C. Weiner[9] lysed red cells by freezing and thawing, precipitated the stroma by incubation of the hemolysate with 50% ethanol at temperatures between −6 and −35 C, and eluted antibody by incubation of the deposit obtained after centrifugation with saline at 37 C. Kochwa and Rosenfield[10] employed digitonin to both lyse red cells and precipitate the stroma. Their procedure, which necessitated the use of high-speed centrifugation to facilitate complete removal of the hemoglobin-stained supernatant, involved elution of antibody into a glycine-HCl buffer at pH 3.0, with subsequent overnight dialysis against buffered saline to restore neutrality.

Apart from aesthetic reasons, hemoglobin-free eluates obviously are not necessary when testing eluates solely by the indirect antiglobulin technique, as in the routine serological evaluation of patients with suspected warm autoimmune hemolytic anemia. For this purpose, Rubin[11] modified the ether elution technique of Vos and Kelsall[5] for use with intact red cells. Minor variations of Rubin's method have been suggested by a number of investigators.

During the past decade, there have been numerous published modifications to the above-mentioned procedures that, according to the authors, permit a considerable reduction in eluate preparation time without significantly reducing the potency of the eluted antibody. Such modifications include the procedure of Jenkins and Moore,[12] which utilizes 0.8 M phosphate buffer at pH 8.2, rather than overnight dialysis, to neutralize the acidic glycine-HCl eluant buffer described by Kochwa and Rosenfield.[10] Other techniques using glycine-HCl buffer at pH 3.0, but with intact red cells as opposed to stroma, have been reported by Rekvig and Hannestad[13] (Appendix 1) and by Bush.[14] The freeze-thaw elution technique of Weiner[9] has been modified to permit elution of anti-A or anti-B from small amounts of red cells obtained from newborn infants with suspected ABO hemolytic disease[15,16] (Appendix 2). Further, alternatives to ether have been used; xylene (Appendix 3) by Chan-Shu and Blair[17] and Bueno et al,[18] and chloroform by Branch et al[19] (Appendix 4).

Alternative methods for dissociation of red cell antigen-antibody complexes continue to be investigated. Hughes-Jones et al[20] have studied the effect of an alkaline pH eluant for the dissociation of anti-D. Edgington[21] investigated the effects of chaotropic ions (Cl^-, I^- and SCN^-), and van Oss et al[22] studied the low surface-energy organic solvent dimethylsulphoxide (DMSO). Such methods do not appear to have much application for routine serological use. However, sonication has been found to be an effective and practical method of elution by both Bird and Wingham,[23] and by Jimerfield[24] (Appendix 5). Finally, Mantel and Holtz[25] reinvestigated some of their earlier work on the effect of quinoline derivatives[26,25] and developed an elution technique using chloroquine diphosphate. This procedure was studied recently by Edwards et al,[28] who noted that chloroquine does not denature red cell antigens, and subsequently developed a method for dissociation of IgG that permits the complete blood group phenotyping of red cells with a positive DAT (Appendix 6).

The Mechanisms of Elution

Three important facets of antigen-antibody reaction hypotheses are worthy of mention when it comes to explaining how elution techniques work. (No definition of terms will be given here, since these have been stated in previous chapters of this book.) First is the law of mass action as it applies to the formation of antigen-antibody complexes, which is generally an exothermic reaction. Second are the electrostatic (Coulombic) and hydrogen bonds, and van der Waals interactions, which hold antigen and antibody together. Third is the need for configurational complementarity between an antigen and its binding site on an antibody molecule. Simply stated, elution methods work by changing the thermodynamics of the antigen-antibody reaction, by neutralizing or reversing forces of attraction, or by disturbing the structural complementarity between antigen and antibody.

Undoubtedly, this is a gross over-simplification. However, it should be stated that there has been considerable debate during the past two decades on precisely how antigen-antibody complexes are formed, and only recently have the factors involved in the reversal of this process received attention. The subject has been reviewed by Howard[29] and to some extent by van Oss et al.[22,30]

Since this author has not been blessed with more than an elementary understanding of physical chemistry, what follows are but a few basic conceptions of how the above-mentioned aspects relating to the mechanisms involved in antigen-antibody reactions might be influenced by the various procedures that have been used to prepare eluates from antibody-coated red cells.

Heat

The generally exothermic reaction for the formation of antigen-antibody complexes can be represented by the equation:

$$(1) \quad Ag + Ab \rightleftharpoons [AgAb] + \text{calories.}[30]$$

Consequently, an increase in temperature can be expected to result in displacement of the equation to the left, or dissociation of [AgAb]. On a molecular level, an increase in heat leads to an increase in the thermal motion of atoms and molecules, resulting in dissociation.[29]

An increase in heat also causes conformational changes to proteins, leading to a loss of structural complementarity between antigen and antibody. Heat at 60 C is detrimental to proteins, and at 56 C denaturation of red cell membranes occurs, as manifested by the hemoglobin-stained appearance of eluates prepared by the Landsteiner and Miller technique.[1] Calvin et al[31] and Lubinski and Portnuff[32] have shown that red cells incubated at 56 C for five minutes are not agglutinated by anti-Rh sera, and the supernatant of a suspension of red cells treated in this manner will inhibit anti-Rh antibodies.[33] Recently, Ballas and Miguel[34] found that membranes isolated from red cells exposed to heat at 50 C for ten minutes gave an abnormal staining pattern following polyacrylamide gel electrophoresis. Fy^a and Jk^a antigens were denatured by such treatment, as were M and P_1 antigens to a lesser degree. Other antigens were not adversely affected. It is unclear precisely what the significance of these observations is, for it will be seen later that heat elution is not optimal for the dissociation of Duffy and Kidd antibodies.

Hapten Addition

The effect of hapten addition to a preformed red cell antigen-antibody complex can be represented by the equation:

$$(2) \quad Hp + AgAb \rightleftharpoons [HpAb] + Ag.$$

This explains how water soluble antigens or sugars can dissociate agglutinates formed by allohemagglutinins or lectins, respectively. However, hapten addition techniques will not be completely effective unless the binding constant of the hapten-antibody interaction is higher than that between red cell antigens and antibodies. Also, hapten may be substituted for antigen in equation (1):

$$(3) \quad Hp + Ab \rightleftharpoons [HpAb] + calories,$$

so that [HpAb] also can be dissociated by physical or chemical means, thereby permitting the recovery of antibody (or lectin) in a useable form.

Freeze-Thawing

As red cells are gradually frozen at below -3 C, extracellular ice crystals are formed which attract pure water from their surroundings. This increases the osmolarity of the remaining extracellular fluid, which then extracts water from the red cells. The red cells shrink, and eventually lysis occurs, probably because of mechanical damage to red cell membranes by the crystals.[35] Some dissociation of antibody might occur as a result of changes to the ionic strength of the extracellular fluid and rearrangement of water molecules at the red cells surface (see effect of chaotropic ions). Disruption of red cell membranes may lead to denaturation of antigens. Also, antigens may actually be shed from rigid red cell membranes[36]; a condition that can be presumed to exist with red cells at subzero temperatures.

However, a considerable amount of antibody must remain on sensitized red cells subjected to the action of freezing and thawing, for this procedure is included as a preparatory step in a number of stromal elution techniques[2,4-9] that utilize other physical manipulations, or chemical means, to dissociate bound antibody. Thus, perhaps the only tenable explanation for the action of the Lui easy-freeze method[16,17] is simply one of conformational changes to membrane structures that

179

occur as a consequence of the dramatic and rapid changes to the ambient temperature of the red cells that is inherent in this technique.

Sonication

High-frequency sound waves cause a very rapid alternation in pressure within fluid media, so that large numbers of minute gas bubbles are formed. As these bubbles grow to a critical size they implode, causing shock waves that exert considerable shearing forces.[23] Simply stated, antibody molecules are shaken off the red cells. Considerable heat is also produced by sonication, and may contribute to the dissociation of bound antibody.

Alterations to pH

At high or low pH levels, all proteins tend to become either negatively charged (anionic state, high pH) or positively charged (cationic state, low pH).[37] Under such conditions, proteins not only lose their ability to attract one another through electrostatic bonding, but may be forced apart by repulsion of similar charges.[29] Positively charged hydrogen ions and negatively charged hydroxyl groups, which abound in low and high pH solutions respectively, are attracted to opposite charges on certain polar aminoacids such as lysine, arginine and histidine (positively charged R groups), and aspartic and glutamic acids (negatively charged R groups). This affects the tertiary structure of proteins by causing molecular unfolding. At extreme alkaline pH levels the secondary structure of proteins may be affected by dissociation of peptide bonds.[29]

Chaotropic Ions at High Concentrations

Chaotropic ions (Cl^-, I^-, SCN^-) literally cause "chaos" to proteins. They bind to charged groups on aminoacids that govern the tertiary structure of proteins (ie, R groups involved with intermolecular bonds). This may lead to molecular unfolding and, perhaps, disruption of peptide bonds.[38,39] At high concentrations, the "salting-out" of proteins occurs, which involves the inward folding of polypeptide chains leading to a decrease in protein solubility.[37,39] High concentrations of salts, therefore, cause conformational changes to the structure of antigens and antibodies.

With respect to the effect of chaotropic ions on the forces involved in the first stage of the hemagglutination reaction, electrostatic shielding of charged groups by counterions leads to weaking of the forces of attraction between antigen and antibody.[30,38] Also, since solutions containing high concentrations of salts can attract water from a place of lower ionic concentration,[35] there may be some rearrangement to the ordered water molecules at the red cell surface. This will undoubtedly influence the "hydrophobic effect" involving van der Waals interactions.[40]

Organic Solvents

Vos and Kelsall[5] speculated that organic solvents such as ether destroy or denature antigens, while antibody molecules are unaffected. Presumably, this might occur by dissolution of the red cell membrane bilipid layer. Other workers[20,41] suggest that ether acts by altering the tertiary structure of antibodies. Either modification would obviously disturb structural complementarity.

Recently, van Oss et al[40,42] showed that attractive forces arising from van der Waals interactions can be changed to forces of repulsion by lowering the surface tension of the liquid medium to a point intermediate between that of the antigen and its binding site on an antibody molecule. While the calculations involved in determining surface tension values and the theory involved are beyond the comprehension of this author, van Oss et al[22] have used the following equations to demonstrate the intent of their experiments:

$$\gamma AgV > \gamma LV > \gamma AbV,$$

where L stands for liquid, V for vapor and γ for surface tension. Although their experiments were performed using DMSO to lower the surface tension of the liquid medium, other organic solvents (eg, ether, chloroform, xylene) probably exert a similar effect.[40]

Chloroquine Diphosphate

The most likely action of this substance appears to be one of neutralization of charges by counterions similar to, but milder than, the effect of chaotropic ions. Evidence for this comes from the studies by Holtz et al,[26] who found red cells suspended in chloroquine to have a reduced electrophoretic mobility. Antigens and antibodies were not denatured, and normal electrophoretic mobility was observed after removal of chloroquine.

ZZAP Reagent

It is to be assumed that the action of ZZAP reagent (a mixture of cysteine-activated papain and dithiothreitol) on antigen-antibody complexes involves both proteolysis of immunoglobulins and cleavage

181

of interchain disulphide bonds. Studies with antisera to fragments of IgG (Fc, Fab, F(ab')$_2$) against IgG coated red cells treated with ZZAP reagent are nonreactive (Branch DR, personal communication). However, these immunoglobulin fragments have not been demonstrated in supernatants obtained after such treatment.

Further Comments

It should be stated that the preceding discussion is highly speculative. Studies to define the action of elution techniques have yet to be performed. Also, any manipulations to a preformed antigen-antibody complex that results in conformational changes to immunoglobulins will only be effective for elution purposes providing that such changes are minimal and reversible (ie, the secondary structure of proteins is not affected). Otherwise, serologically inactive eluates will be obtained.

Factors That Influence the Outcome of Elution Techniques

Technical Considerations

Specific details of some of the more commonly employed elution techniques are to be found at the end of this chapter, and will not be discussed in any depth here. However, those procedures given in the AABB *Technical Manual*[43] (heat, ether, digitonin-acid) are not included in the Appendices. What follows is a discussion of some of the technical factors that influence the success of elution studies and how some of the pitfalls of antibody elution from red cells may be avoided.

Incomplete Washing

To ensure that the antibody activity of an eluate is red cell membrane derived, and does not represent residual serum antibody activity, thorough washing of the red cells prior to elution is essential. Six washes are usually more than adequate, but further washes may be necessary when red cells have been sensitized with a high-titer antibody in vitro. As a means of controlling the efficacy of the washing process it is appropriate to test the supernatant solution, obtained from the final wash phase, for antibody activity in parallel with the eluate.

On rare occasions, however, the presence of antibody activity in the final wash solution may not be necessarily the result of inadequate

182

washing of the antibody-coated red cells. Such a misleading finding may occur when dealing with low-affinity antibodies that readily dissociate at room temperature.

Binding of Proteins to Glass Surfaces

If eluates are prepared from red cells coated with high-titer antibodies in vitro, and the same test tube that was used during the sensitization phase is also used for preparing the eluate, antibody that has become bound nonspecifically to the test tube surface may dissociate during the elution phase, leading to contamination of the eluate. To avoid such contamination, it is appropriate to transfer the red cells during the washing phase into a clean test tube before proceeding with the preparation of the eluate.

Storage Changes to Organic Solvents

Organic solvents, particularly ether, become acidic during storage, probably as the result of peroxide formation. This may account for the apparent "nonspecific" activity of eluates when ether has been used from an almost empty canister (Beattie KM, personal communication). Consequently, it is advisable to discard organic solvents when the container is one-quarter full.

Dissociation of Antibody Prior to Elution

This is not usually a problem with IgG antibodies unless they have a low affinity for their respective red cell antigens. It may, however, contribute to the difficulties encountered when attempting to elute cold reactive antibodies such as autoanti-I, anti-M and the polyagglutinins (anti-T, anti-Tn, etc). To minimize the loss of antibody during the wash phase, the use of cold (4 C) saline is recommended.

Incorrect Technique

Depending upon the elution method used, such factors as incomplete removal of organic solvents and failure to render the eluate isotonic or to a neutral pH, may result in the red cells used to test the eluate either hemolyzing or appearing "sticky." Similarly, the presence of stromal debris in an eluate may interfere with the reading of tests. Careful technique and strict adherence to method protocols will help mitigate such problems.

183

Stability of Eluates

Dilute protein solutions, such as are obtained in eluates other than those prepared directly into serum or albumin, are unstable. Therefore, it is good practice to test eluates as soon after preparation as possible. Alternatively, if protein is added in the form of bovine albumin to a final concentration of 6% (w/v), eluates may be kept frozen for several months and still retain their antibody activity.

Nonspecific Attachment of Immunoglobulins to Red Cells

The Matuhasi-Ogata Phenomenon

Matuhasi[44] showed that when group A Rh-negative red cells were agglutinated by an anti-A serum that also contained anti-D, both anti-A (right antibody) and anti-D (wrong antibody) could be recovered in eluates prepared from those red cells. Also, Matuhasi and colleagues[45] found that both anti-A (right) and anti-B (wrong) could be eluted from group A red cells that had been preincubated with anti-A and then subsequently incubated with anti-B. The terms "right" and "wrong" were introduced by Allen et al[46] to denote the specific and nonspecific uptake of antibody by the adsorbing red cells, respectively. Further, Ogata and Matuhasi[47,48] showed that agglutination of red cells was not necessary for the phenomenon to occur, that both IgG and IgM immunoglobulins could bind other antibodies nonspecifically, and that the phenomenon occurred with mixtures of antibody-containing sera, as well as individual sera containing multiple antibody specificities.

As originally described, the Matuhasi-Ogata phenomenon was considered to be the nonspecific uptake of antibody molecules by a preformed immune complex. The observations of Svardal et al[49] and Allen et al[46] have been attributed to this phenomenon. Both groups of investigators found that alloantibodies, directed towards antigens not present on the adsorbing red cells, could be recovered in eluates when the adsorbing red cells were from patients with autoimmune hemolytic anemia. In 45 different experiments, using red cells incubated with alloantibodies in vitro, Allen et al[46] were either able to recover the wrong antibody by elution, or demonstrate its partial removal by titration of the adsorbed serum, in 31 cases (69% of total tests). The Matuhasi-Ogata phenomenon, per se, also has been used to explain the loss of desired antibody activity when typing reagents are adsorbed to remove unwanted isohemagglutinins,[46] and to explain the findings of Dunsford and Stapleton,[50] who were able to adsorb weak anti-D antibodies onto autologous Rh-negative red cells that had become coated with anti-I when whole blood samples were maintained at 4 C.

Cytophilic IgG

Boursnell et al[51] showed that all red cells are coated with IgG nonimmunologically, and estimates of the amount of IgG that is bound to red cells in this fashion (cytophilic IgG) are as high as 200,000 molecules per red cell.[52] Gergely et al[53,54] have shown that cytophilic IgG comprises a distinct population of immunoglobulin molecules that are resistant to cleavage by papain in the absence of cysteine, and it has been suggested[51] that cytophilic IgG is bound differently on red cells (ie, the Fc fragment is not oriented in the correct manner for binding with anti-IgG) to that bound by a specific antigen-antibody interaction. Such a conclusion is, of course, essential in order that the interpretation of the mechanism of the antiglobulin test is not compromised.

In attempting to explain the Matuhasi-Ogata phenomenon as a manifestation of cytophilic IgG, Bove et al[55] used ^{125}I-labeled antibodies of various specificities in conjunction with ^{131}I-labeled IgG that was devoid of antibody activity. They found the amount of IgG (in addition to that already present) that could be bound nonimmunologically was as high as 17,500 molecules per red cell. Also, they showed that when a high-titer anti-D was incubated with Rh-negative red cells, the amount of serologically active IgG bound nonimmunologically, although only a small fraction of the total cytophilic IgG, was sufficient to result in the detection of anti-D in eluates prepared from those red cells. Further, they found that red cells precoated with IgG by a specific antigen-antibody interaction would adsorb as much IgG nonimmunologically as unsensitized red cells. This latter observation is not consistent with the uptake of antibodies by preformed immune complexes (Matuhasi-Ogata phenomenon).

Further Observations

It may seem that two distinct phenomena (Matuhasi-Ogata and cytophilic IgG) can account for the nonspecific adsorption of antibodies by red cells. That this is not necessarily the case is apparent from the studies of McKeever.[56] Her studies revealed that wrong antibody could be adsorbed by red cells even in the absence of a preformed antigen-antibody complex. However, the frequency with which such nonspecific adsorption occurred (23% of experiments) was less than when the adsorbing red cells were presensitized with a specific antibody (44% of experiments). She found a number of factors influenced the degree and, therefore, the recognition of this nonspecific binding. These factors included temperature (4 C better than 37 C), and precoating the red cells with drug (particularly cephalothin) or complement potentiated the phenomenon. Detection of the wrong antibody by elution was enhanced when eluates were prepared into a protein medium as opposed to saline, and the presence of the wrong antibody was more frequently observed when heat eluates were prepared than when Rubin's ether technique[11] was used. Finally, there was not an increase in nonspecific adsorption when the serum:red cell ratio was increased tenfold, or when enzyme-pretreated red cells were used.

Significance to the Serologist

There are a number of circumstances in which the nonspecific adsorption of immunoglobulins by red cells may impact on the outcome of eluate test results. First, it should be understood that when an eluate is prepared from red cells of an alloimmunized patient with concomitant autoantibodies the reactivity of that eluate may not solely represent autoantibody (ie, alloantibody may also be present). Second, when attempting to isolate individual alloantibodies from a multispecific serum by selective adsorption and elution tests, the wrong antibody (directed towards an antigen not present on the adsorbing red cells) may be recovered in the eluate. Third, as shown by Wilkinson et al,[57] false-positive eluate test results (as well as false-positive D^u tests) may occur if anti-D sera containing anti-Bg antibodies are used to test Rh-negative, Bg-positive red cells. Similar findings can be expected to occur when using antisera containing other contaminating antibodies to low-incidence red cell antigens.

It might be inferred, from what has already been discussed, that the nonimmunological adsorption of immunoglobulins by red cells invalidates the result of all combined adsorption-elution experiments. However, as stated by Issitt and Issitt,[58 (p 346)] this is not so in practice. Often the wrong antibody in eluates is present in such low levels that it goes undetected and when it is observed, it is always present in much smaller quantities than the right antibody so that it can be easily recognized as not being the part of a specific antigen-antibody interaction. Nonetheless, some caution is necessary when performing critical studies as, for example, in the separation of two antibodies, such as anti-En[a] and anti-Wr[b], where a double adsorption-elution procedure may be used to ensure the purity of eluate preparations.[59]

Finally, the effect of cytophilic IgG in the quantitative estimation of the antibody content of eluates has been studied recently by Masouredis et al.[60] Using ^{125}I-labeled anti-D, they found the specific radioactivity of digitonin-acid eluates from Rh-positive red cells to be significantly (80-95%) less than that of the ^{125}I-labeled anti-D IgG used to sensitize the red cells. They attribute this discrepancy to the release of unlabeled cytophilic IgG from normal red cells during eluate preparation, rather than an underestimation of the eluate anti-D content. Further, they found that the presence of cytophilic IgG in an eluate reduces the nonspecific-binding of serologically active IgG. They conclude that their observations justify the assumption that the specific radioactivity of ^{125}I-labeled IgG fractions can be used to provide a valid estimate of the anti-D content of eluates.

Sensitivity of Elution Procedures

Concentration Effect

Despite the claims of some investigators[61] that there is an appreciable loss of antibody during a combined adsorption-elution procedure, this is not the case. We have shown (Judd WJ, et al, unpublished observations) that the sensitivity of the conventional antiglobulin test is such that the lowest level of anti-D that can be detected with reliability is in the order of 0.005 μg/ml. This figure is in agreement with that quoted by Mollison.[62 (p 461)] Extrapolating figures from calculations previously published by Judd and Jenkins,[63] a serum concentration of 0.005 μg/ml of anti-D corresponds to 2×10^{10} molecules of IgG per ml. If 5 ml of this serum are mixed with 1 ml of packed $R_1 R_1$ red cells (1 $\times$ 10^{10} red cells; 20,000 D sites per red cell), a situation of considerable antigen excess will exist (2×10^{14} D sites, 1×10^{11} molecules of anti-D IgG), and virtually all anti-D molecules might be expected to be bound to the red cells. Subsequently, when an eluate is prepared from those red cells into 1 ml of eluant, and assuming that there is a maximum recovery of 80% of the bound antibody, the eluate can be expected to contain 8×10^{10} molecules, or 0.02 μg/ml of anti-D IgG; a figure readily detectable by the antiglobulin test. That is to say the reactivity of the eluate will be about four times stronger than that of the native serum. Obviously, even more potent eluates can be obtained by increasing the serum:red cell ratio used in the sensitization phase prior to elution or by reducing the volume of the eluant.

Potentiation Effect

The above experiment and calculations can also be applied to explain why sometimes it is possible to obtain a serologically reactive eluate from red cells with a negative DAT. Incubation of 1×10^{10} red cells with 1×10^{11} molecules of IgG antibody will result in each red cell being coated with approximately ten antibody molecules. This figure is well below the threshold of detection for the antiglobulin test, which is in the order of 150 to 500 molecules of IgG per red cell.[62 (p 443)] When three volumes of eluate prepared from these red cells are incubated with one volume of a 4% suspension of antigen-positive red cells, as in the conventional antiglobulin test, the number of antibody molecules that may be bound to each red cell will be $(3 \times 8 \times 10^{10} \times n) \div (0.04 \times 10^{10} \times n)$ (where n = the size of the drop volumes used), or 600 molecules of IgG per red cell; a level sufficient for detection by antiglobulin serum. In this case, it is not simply the fact that antibody has been concentrated by elution that permits its detection. Rather, the molecular concentrations of the reactants in the test phase are such that they afford a much greater uptake of antibody by the test red cells compared to that originally present on the red cells from which the eluate was prepared.

Classical situations in which red cells with a negative DAT test may yield a reactive eluate due to this potentiation effect are ABO hemolytic disease of the newborn[64,65] and some cases of warm autoimmune hemolytic anemia.[66 (p 305)] However, in ABO hemolytic disease of the newborn there is evidence that suggests IgG anti-A/B molecules are bound to the infant's red cells in a manner that is not conducive for binding with anti-IgG, rather than simply being present in low levels.[64,67] When eluates are prepared and incubated with adult group A or group B red cells, the antibody molecules are bound in the correct fashion to yield a positive antiglobulin test.

Elution Studies in the Evaluation of Blood Samples with a Positive DAT

The evaluation of blood samples with a positive DAT is an important function of a blood bank, and the significance of such a finding should be familiar to most readers of this article. Detailed reviews of the causes of a positive DAT and the specificities of autoantibodies have been published by the American Association of Blood Banks,[68,69] and by others.[66,70,71] Briefly, a positive test in the neonate usually is associated with hemolytic disease of the newborn induced by maternal antibodies, and in other patients a positive test may be associated with autoimmune hemolytic anemia or drug therapy. In recently transfused individuals, a positive test may result from the passive transfer of

188

antibody (eg, when group O platelet concentrates, containing anti-A and anti-B, are administered to a group A, B or AB recipient), or may be indicative of alloimmune hemolytic anemia. The latter condition should be of considerable concern to the blood banker, for it results from the transfusion of either frankly incompatible blood or (hopefully, more usually) from a delayed immune response to the transfusion of what were seemingly serologically compatible red cells.

Routine Testing of Eluates

It is important that the routine serological procedures (including elution studies) employed in the evaluation of blood samples with a positive DAT are capable of differentiating the above causes of immune red cell destruction. Also, in conjunction with these studies, it is important to obtain a detailed summary of the patient's diagnosis, drug therapy and transfusion history. Such information is invaluable when attempting to interpret the serological data obtained. Further, it should be remembered that the results of serological tests are not diagnostic, and their significance can only be assessed in light of the clinical condition of the patient concerned. Thus, other laboratory data (eg, bilirubin, haptoglobin, hematocrit, reticulocyte count) are required before the clinical significance of serological findings can be determined.

Neonatal Blood Samples

Studies on cord blood samples to diagnose hemolytic disease of the newborn should be directed primarily towards the recognition of maternally derived antibody in the eluate. This may necessitate the use of a panel of phenotyped group O reagent red cells, and the use of groups A or B red cells in the diagnosis of ABO hemolytic disease of the newborn. When no antibody is apparent in the maternal sample, testing the eluate against the father's red cells is appropriate to establish that the cause of the positive DAT is due to a fetal-maternal incompatibility. This apparent lack of maternal antibody is likely to be encountered when the father's red cells carry a low-incidence blood group antigen that is not represented among the reagent red cell panel samples.

Further use of the eluate may be of value in selection of blood for exchange transfusion. Such usage is appropriate when a maternal blood sample is unavailable, or when the maternal serum contains multiple alloantibodies, such as anti-Le^{a+b} and anti-Fy^a. Only the latter antibody is of concern in this situation, for it is well known that

Lewis antibodies do not cause hemolytic disease of the newborn and should not be present in the eluate.[47(p 276)] Thus, it is not only time-consuming but inappropriate to select Le(a−b−), Fy(a−) units for exchange transfusion based on their compatibility with the maternal serum. Rather, Fy(a−) units, regardless of their Lewis phenotype, may be selected and crossmatched with the eluate prepared from the cord blood red cells.

All Other Samples

The routine testing of eluates prepared from blood samples other than those obtained from neonates should ensure the recognition of warm-reactive autoantibodies, passively acquired antibodies, alloantibodies made in response to a recent blood transfusion and antibodies made following therapy with penicillin and cephalothin. Initially, it is appropriate to test the eluate against a panel of phenotyped group O reagent red cells, and to include tests with enzyme-treated red cells. To ensure the detection of weak examples of autoantibodies and weakly reactive examples of Rh, Kell and Kidd antibodies that may be made in response to transfusion, three enzyme-treated red cell samples should be used. These should be of the phenotypes $R_1 R_1$, $R_2 R_2$ and rr, and include among them one K+ sample, one Jk(a+b−), and one Jk(a−b+).

Further Diagnostic Studies

Depending upon the results obtained during the initial testing, further studies may be necessary. For example, if an alloantibody is present, additional examples of red cells of the relevant phenotype should be used to confirm specificity. If these initial tests are nonreactive, and if the patient's medical history so indicates, tests with penicillin- and cephalothin-coated red cells, prepared in the manner described by Garratty,[72] or tests with group A and B red cells to detect passively acquired allohemagglutinins resulting from the infusion of non-ABO-type specific blood products, should be undertaken. Identification of autoantibody specificity is often of only academic interest, but may be of limited value when the patient is actively hemolyzing and must be transfused. In this situation, titration of the eluate and testing each dilution against $R_1 R_1$, $R_2 R_2$ and rr red cells may permit the recognition of an anti-Rh-like antibody (eg, anti-e-like). In such a circumstance, the transfusion of $R_2 R_2$ (e-negative) blood may be of some benefit to the patient concerned.[66(p 372),73] However, the testing of all eluates containing warm-reactive autoantibodies against such exotic red cells as Rh_{null} and D-deletion phenotypes is not advocated. Rarely would such blood be available for transfusion, if that should prove necessary. Indeed, it would be an inappropriate use of rare donor units. Further, the knowledge that an autoantibody fails to react with red cells of these uncommon phenotypes is of little value to the physician in the clinical management of the patient.

The Appropriateness of Performing Elution Studies on Pretransfusion Samples

We recently reported (Judd et al[74]) the incidence of a positive DAT in our institution to be as high as 15% of samples submitted to our blood bank for routine pretransfusion testing. This percentage is at variance with the incidence reported in separate studies by Worledge[75] (8% of patients) and Freedman[76] (7% of patients). The plethora of samples requiring evaluation, which included elution studies, caused us to focus our attention on those patients with a positive DAT who were either anemic for reasons other than blood loss or who had been transfused within the previous three weeks, and those whose serum contained unexpected antibodies.

The results of a retrospective analysis on 879 blood samples from patients that met our criteria are shown in group 1 of Table 1. Only 81 reactive eluates were obtained (9% of samples studied). Sixty-four eluates contained autoantibodies, three contained antibody to penicillin-coated red cells and another three contained passively acquired anti-A. The remaining 11 reactive eluates contained alloantibodies made in response to a recent transfusion. In six (55%) of the latter samples the transfusion-induced alloantibody was not detected in the serum.

It is our contention that the incorporation of the DAT in pretransfusion studies should be used primarily to detect alloantibody formation in response to a recent transfusion, before such antibodies are evident in the serum. In this regard, meaningful data was obtained by elution in six (0.68%) of the 879 samples studied. Also, all but one of the transfusion-induced alloantibodies were detected within 14 days of transfusion, and only one of 389 samples in which complement (C3) alone was present on the red cells yielded an alloantibody upon elution. Consequently, we have refined our policies, and elution studies are now restricted (apart from diagnostic testing for autoimmune hemolytic anemia) to those blood samples from patients who have been transfused within the past two weeks. Further, an anti-IgG reagent, as opposed to a polyspecific (anti-IgG+C3) antiglobulin serum, is now used when performing the pretransfusion DAT.

Table 1.—Results of Elution Studies on Pretransfusion Blood Samples with a Positive Direct Antiglobulin Test (University of Michigan Data)

	Group 1	Group 2
Time period	8 months, 1978	24 months, 1980-81
Pretransfusion samples	12,187	46,672
Positive tests	1,839	2,572
Samples evaluated	879*	480†
Reactive eluates - total	81	152
- auto	64	111
- passive	3	0
- penicillin	3	8
- allo	11 (6)‡	33 (5)‡

*Samples from patients with suspected hemolysis, or transfused within previous three weeks or with unexpected serum antibodies. Positive direct antiglobulin tests obtained with a polyspecific antiglobulin reagent.
† Samples from patients transfused within previous two weeks. Positive direct antiglobulin tests obtained with an anti-IgG reagent.
‡ Figure in parenthesis denotes number of alloantibodies detected only by elution.

Under our present criteria, 33 transfusion-induced alloantibodies were encountered among 480 eluates prepared during 1980-81 (group 2 of Table 1). In contrast to our earlier study, all but five (15%) of alloantibodies were detected in the serum as well as in the eluate. This may be attributed to the use of low-ionic strength saline (LISS) in screening tests for unexpected antibodies during 1980-81, as opposed to saline-albumin tests in 1978.

Comments on the Interpretation of Eluate Test Results

An in-depth discussion of the serological findings that may be encountered in the evaluation of blood samples with a positive DAT is beyond the scope of this chapter. The interested reader is referred elsewhere[66,68-71] for detailed reviews and references to original articles on the specificities of the antibodies involved. However, two situations in which differentiation between allo- and autoantibody cannot readily be made are worthy of mention.

Autoantibodies Mimicking Alloantibodies

The specificity of an antibody eluted from the red cells of a patient with a positive DAT may not, on occasion, correlate with the phenotype of those red cells (ie, the "wrong" antibody is eluted). Invariably, the antibody in question is also present as "free antibody" in the serum, and in light of the lack of corresponding antigen on the patient's red cells may be concluded (incorrectly) as being an alloantibody. However, that this is not the case can be shown by adsorption and elution studies; the antibody can be adsorbed by, and subsequently eluted from, antigen-negative red cells, which is quite unlike the behavior of an alloantibody.

This phenomenon was first reported by Fudenberg et al[77] in 1958. According to Petz and Garratty,[66(p 246)] anti-E eluted from E-negative red cells is by far the most common "wrong" antibody seen. Other specificities, including anti-c and anti-E,[78] anti-C,[79] and anti-K[60,80] have been reported.

In the case described by Fudenberg et al, it was suggested that the antibody might be reacting with all antigens containing a basic Rh structure, but which preferentially bound to one or more specific Rh determinants. A similar hypothesis was proposed by Rosenfield (cited in reference 78) who, in commenting on an example of "mimicking" anti-E, suggested that the immunoglobulin producing cells of the patient might be making a population of antibody molecules with a poorly differentiated specificity that were capable of binding more readily to E-positive than to E-negative red cells.

In discussing these autoantibodies that mimic alloantibodies, it is not possible to avoid returning to the Matuhasi-Ogata phenomenon for an explanation, although this seems unlikely. Issitt and Issitt[58(p 347)] have invoked the term "Super" Matuhasi-Ogata to classify the recovery of large quantities of wrong antibody bound in vivo, and contrast it to the Matuhasi-Ogata "minimus" condition when only small amounts of wrong antibody are recovered during in vitro adsorption-elution experiments. Issitt et al[78] consider the "minimus" condition to result from cytophilic IgG.

Alloantibodies Mimicking Autoantibodies

Although not a common occurrence, alloantibodies to high-incidence red cell antigens (eg, anti-U, anti-hr^B) may be encountered in red cell eluates (and serum) from recently transfused individuals. On initial testing, the serological results obtained are often indistinguishable from those associated with warm-reactive autoantibodies. In order to recognize the potential for alloantibody involvement, the need for a detailed patient history cannot be over emphasized.

Contrary to what has been stated regarding the identification of autoantibodies, additional tests for alloantibody recognition and identification are mandatory when the patient has been transfused recently, and especially so when no previous autoantibody involvement has been documented. Additional eluate (and/or serum) studies should include tests with red cells lacking high-incidence antigens. However, these studies may not be diagnostic, and the utilization of procedures beyond the scope of this chapter (eg, studies on autologous red cells isolated by differential centrifugation through phthalate ester mixtures[43(p 416)]) may be required to ensure the satisfactory resolution of such complex serological problems.

Applications of Adsorption-Elution Tests

One has only to read any standard text book on immunohematology to appreciate how much information concerning the intricacies of the blood group phenotypes has been gathered exclusively by the use of combined adsorption-elution studies. The data obtained include the recognition of the para-Bombay and dominant Lu(a−b−) phenotypes,[81,82] the recognition of anti-G as a component of some anti-CD sera,[83] and the complexities of anti-KL and anti-En[a] antibodies.[59,84,85] While this information is sometimes only of academic interest, adsorption and elution tests are extremely informative, if not mandatory, when applied to the confirmation of antigens with a low-site density or the detection of weakly reactive antibodies. Also, they may be invaluable in the separation of antibody mixtures for identification or reagent production purposes. In this section, some practical and theoretical aspects of these and other applications of combined adsorption-elution tests, beyond those previously mentioned, will be discussed.

Detection of Weak Antigens and Antibodies

Adsorption of antibody, to demonstrate the presence or absence of the corresponding antigen on red cells, is best accomplished using a low serum to red cells ratio (eg, 2:1 or less). Care should be taken not to dilute the serum (and hence the antibody) with residual saline from inadequately packed red cells, and the determination of the protein concentrations of the pre- and postadsorbed serum by refractometry is an appropriate check for such dilution. A reduction in titration score of ten or more (using the scoring system described by Marsh[86]) following a threefold adsorption is considered significant evidence for the presence of the relevant antigen on the adsorbing red cells. In critical studies, control adsorptions with red cells known to lack the antigen in question should be undertaken.

Since eluates are likely to yield more antibody when a high serum:red cell ratio is used (eg, 5:1 or more), it is advisable to perform a combined adsorption-elution procedure in two stages; using significantly more serum than red cells during the sensitization phase prior to elution, and a lower ratio during subsequent adsorptions. Testing an aliquot of unsensitized red cells from the same sample used in these studies against the eluate can be of value in showing whether or not the antibody was subject to elution.

Identification of Antibodies in Multispecific Sera

Adsorption-elution studies may be used for identification purposes with sera containing multiple antibodies. Since these studies are tedious, they should be undertaken when all other tests, including studies with multiple reagent red cell samples and tests with enzyme-pretreated cells, have failed to resolve the problem fully. Availability of sufficient quantities of red cells is essential, and the phenotyping of staff members is invaluable.

The choice of adsorbing red cells is of great importance to the success of these studies, but often has to be an inspired guess; influenced by the phenotype of the antibody producer. Knowing which alloantibodies could be present should lead the technologist to focus attention on proving their presence or absence. As a general rule, one or more of the weakly reactive red cell samples should be used, on the assumption that these will carry only one of the factors to which the serum has specificity.

The serum under investigation should be adsorbed several times, until it no longer reacts with the adsorbing red cells. An eluate, prepared from the red cells used in the first adsorption, and the adsorbed serum, should then be examined for antibody specificity. While it is to be hoped that specific antibodies will be apparent in either or both preparations, this is not always the case. Some antibodies are difficult to adsorb and elute (eg, the so-called high-titer, low-avidity antibodies—anti-Kn^a, etc). Also, the adsorbed serum may be nonreactive, yet the eluate reacts with all reagent cell samples. Such a finding may indicate the presence of an antibody to a high-incidence antigen that has a variable expression on red cells, or may be due to the fact that one is dealing with a weakly reactive antibody that was subject to dilution during the adsorption process.

When the above studies are not informative, or when autoantibodies are present in the serum of a recently transfused individual so that an autologous adsorption is not appropriate, selective adsorptions with R_1R_1, R_2R_2 and rr red cells may be helpful in the identification of alloantibodies. Beattie[87] recommends that all three red cell samples used for this purpose be K−, and include among them one Jk(a−), one Jk(b−) and another Fy(a−). The adsorbed serum samples, and eluates prepared from the red cells used in the first adsorption, are then examined for antibody specificity.

Isolation of Specific Antibodies

Antibodies of desired specificities can be isolated from sera containing unwanted allohemagglutinins and other contaminating antibodies by adsorption with, and subsequent elution from, red cells of the appropriate phenotype. For example, if group A red cells are to be typed for Xg^a and the only example of anti-Xg^a is from a group O donor, eluates prepared from group O Xg(a+) red cells preincubated with the serum will contain anti-Xg^a devoid of allohemagglutinins. This is also an effective way of preparing rare antisera to high-incidence antigens for use with red cells of all ABO phenotypes, since groups A and B (or AB) red cells lacking the relevant antigen are unlikely to be available for the purpose of removing the allohemagglutinins by adsorption. For aesthetic reasons, hemoglobin-free eluates prepared by the digitonin-acid elution technique are to be preferred when purifying antibodies in this manner for reagent use.

The same approach can be applied to confirm the specificity of serological reactions, particularly when a serum is seen to react with a number of reagent red cell samples that do not appear to share a common antigen. Such findings may be due to the presence of several antibodies to low-incidence antigens, or a single antibody to an unknown determinant (ie, one that the reagent red cell samples have not been tested for). In the latter instance, an eluate prepared after incubation of the test serum with one of the reactive red cell samples will be seen to react with all the other red cells to which the test serum originally displayed activity.

Further Applications of Elution

Purification of Lectins

While lectins may be isolated in pure form by any conventional protein purification technique, virtually all contemporary methods employ a process known as affinity chromatography, which exploits the sugar-binding capacity of lectins. A crude lectin preparation is passed over a column of an insolubilized carbohydrate ligand (eg, chitin, Sepharose) with which the lectin interacts. Displacement of the bound lectin is accomplished by elution with either a sugar that competes for binding sites with the specific adsorbent or by changing the pH or ionic strength of the eluant.[88]

A modification of this process, involving the use of red cells as the adsorbent, has been described by Anstee et al[89] for the purification of the peanut lectin, *Arachis hypogea* (anti-T). T-activated, formaldehyde-treated red cells were incubated with a saline extract of the lectin. The red cells were washed to remove unbound protein, and the lectin dissociated by the addition of 0.15 M lactose. The supernatant fluid obtained after centrifugation was dialyzed extensively against distilled water to remove lactose and then lyophilized.

Obtaining Antibody-Free Intact Red Cells

Sometimes the serologist is required to remove antibody from red cells without causing drastic alteration to the integrity of the red cell membranes. The primary objective of such methods is not necessarily to recover the bound antibody in a useable form but, rather, to obtain antibody-free red cells for use in further testing.

Dispersal of Cold Autoagglutination

In CHD the autologous red cells tend to agglutinate spontaneously, and the preparation of a red cell suspension for typing purposes may be difficult. Often this can be accomplished by simple incubation and repeated washing of the red cells with warm (45 C) saline. Alternatively, exposure of the red cells to 56 C heat for three minutes can be used without denaturing red cell antigens. These methods may not, however, be effective when dealing with potent cold-reactive autoagglutinins. In such a situation, thiol reagents which cleave the interchain disulphide bonds of IgM molecules may be used. Reid[90] has described such a procedure, which involves the incubation of equal volumes of red cells and 0.1 M 2-mercaptoethanol or 0.01 M dithiothreitol for ten minutes at 37 C, and found these thiol reagents do not denature antigens of the major blood group systems.

Dissociation of Allohemagglutination

On occasion, it may be necessary to separate mixed populations of red cells (eg, ABO mixtures). Depending upon the type of antisera used, a number of different approaches can be applied to disperse the population of agglutinated red cells. If IgM allohemagglutinins have been used, thiol reagents can be employed as described above. The agglutinated red cells also may be dispersed by the addition of large volumes of group specific substance in the form of ABH secretor saliva. When lectins such as *Dolichos biflorus* (anti-A$_1$) and *Phaseolus limensis* (anti-A) have been used in the red cell separation procedure, agglutination may be dispersed with group A specific substance, or by the addition of the sugar for which these lectins are specific (ie, α-N-acetyl-D-galactosamine). IgG anti-A or anti-B immunoglobulin molecules, which may be present in some commercially prepared ABO typing reagents, are not readily neutralized by soluble blood group substances and their use for separating mixed populations of red cells of differing ABO phenotypes should be avoided if an antibody-free preparation of the agglutinable red cell population is required.

Dissociation of Immune Complexes with Chloroquine Diphosphate

Quinoline derivatives are known to split immune complexes and to inhibit antigen-antibody reactions.[25-27] A procedure for the preparation of eluates from red cells coated in vivo with warm-reactive autoantibodies, involving the use of chloroquine diphosphate, has been described.[25] However, this is not a practical method of elution for routine serological use. Noting that red cell antigens were not denatured following dissociation of IgG by chloroquine diphosphate, Edwards et al[28] developed a method for dissociation of IgG from red cells with a positive DAT that permits subsequent phenotyping of those red cells with antisera solely reactive by the indirect antiglobulin test. This procedure, described in detail in Appendix 6, is of value when investigating blood samples containing both warm-reactive autoantibodies and IgG alloantibodies, since phenotyping these samples for antigens such as Duffy and Kidd cannot otherwise be accomplished except by showing loss of antibody activity following adsorption of the appropriate typing reagent.

Briefly, the procedure involves room temperature incubation of the test red cells in a 20% (w/v) solution of chloroquine diphosphate at pH 5.1, and periodic checking of the DAT with an anti-IgG reagent, for complement components are not dissociated. Edwards et al[28] found that the red cells from 83% of cases involving warm-reactive autoantibodies could be rendered DAT-negative within two hours of treatment. Other samples were less susceptible to dissociation of IgG. In some instances, prolongation of the incubation time or incubation at 37 C may be required for complete dissociation of IgG (Judd WJ, unpublished observations). However, this often causes hemolysis of red cells, and some weakening of Rh antigens. Nonetheless, total loss of Rh antigens does not occur, and the red cells can be typed with modified-tube anti-Rh sera using the indirect antiglobulin technique.

Alloantibodies, used to coat red cells in vitro, are more difficult to dissociate than autoantibodies bound to red cells in vivo.[28]

ZZAP Technique

Branch and Petz[91] found that autoantibodies could be completely dissociated from red cells by incubation with a mixture of cysteine-activated papain and dithiothreitol (ZZAP) reagent. As with all techniques utilizing proteolytic enzymes, ZZAP-treated red cells lack M, N, S and Duffy antigens. In addition, all Kell-system antigens except Kx are denatured by ZZAP. These findings impose considerable limitations on the use of ZZAP-treated red cells for phenotyping purposes. However, enzyme-treated antibody-free red cells for autologous adsorption of sera containing autoantibodies can be obtained less arduously than when the procedure described by Morel[92] is used.

DMSO Technique

Using a mixture of 47.5% (w/v) DMSO and 0.1% bovine albumin at pH 9.0, van Oss et al[22] were able to completely dissociate anti-A, anti-D and anti-K antibodies from sensitized red cells. After incubation of the red cells in alkaline DMSO at 37 C for 30 mintes, followed by centrifugation and removal of the supernatant solution, 2% bovine albumin in pH 7.0 phosphate-buffered saline was added to the red cells under constant agitation on a vortex mixer. Providing the addition of the bovine albumin was carried out slowly until the DMSO concentration was less than 1%, approximately 10% of the original red cells were recovered intact. These red cells were shown to have still retained their A, D and K antigens. Antibody activity was demonstrable in the supernatant after removal of DMSO by overnight dialysis at 4 C.

Placental Eluates

Moulds et al[93] modified the digitonin-acid elution technique of Jenkins and Moore[12] for the recovery of large quantities of antibody from the placental tissue of sensitized women. Their procedure involves homogenization of fresh, unfixed placental tissue in the presence of digitonin, washing the precipitate to remove unbound antibody, elution with pH 3.0 glycine-HCl buffer and subsequent restoration of the eluant to a neutral pH with 0.8 M phosphate buffer at pH 8.0. Approximately one liter of antibody-containing fluid can be recovered by this procedure.

Elution Tests in Forensic Medicine

Since this subject is discussed in depth in another chapter of this book, only some brief comments will be made here. Suffice it to say that fixation-elution techniques are employed by forensic scientists to detect antigens on blood-stained material. Usually, a small (1 cm^2) portion of material is incubated overnight with a specific antibody. The material is washed to remove unbound antibody, incubated in saline at 60 C (elution phase), and the appropriate indicator red cells added and subsequently examined for agglutination. Lincoln and Dodd,[94] have described a micro-elution technique, which incorporates the indirect antiglobulin test for the detection of eluted antibody, that permits the detection of S, s, K, Duffy and Kidd antigens from very small pieces (a single 1 cm strand for each test) of blood-stained material.

Considerations in the Selection of Elution Methods

The selection of a particular elution technique for routine serological use is often one of personal preference, influenced by simplicity of the method and governed by availability of the necessary reagents. From a personal viewpoint, heat elution is best reserved for the investigation of ABO hemolytic disease of the newborn and the elution of predominantly coldreactive antibodies (eg, anti-A/B, anti-I, anti-M). The Lui easy-freeze method (Appendix 2) and sonication (Appendix 5) would appear to be acceptable alternatives. In this author's experience, few other procedures compare (in terms of the amount of reactive antibody eluted) with the technique of Rubin,[11] or modifications thereof, for the elution of IgG auto- and alloantibodies. However, these comments are anecdotal, and undoubtedly differ from the opinions of other investigators. In this section, some more definitive factors in the selection of elution techniques will be discussed.

Eluate Preparation Time

Perhaps one of the major reasons why some of the earlier described elution techniques have not been popularized is the length of time involved in eluate preparation. The procedures described by Komninos and Rosenthal[4] and Kochwa and Rosenfield[10] both involve dialysis of the eluate prior to testing, thus extending the time taken to complete the technique to beyond 24 hours. Also, the methods of Greenwalt[6] and Weiner[9] have been reported to take at least three hours to complete.[95] Among the earlier described procedures, only the techniques of Landsteiner and Miller[1] and Vos and Kelsall[5] can be accomplished within two hours.

Of the techniques included in the Appendices of this chapter and the AABB *Technical Manual*,[43] the quickest (and simplest) is the sonication procedure of Jimerfield.[24] Rubin's elution technique[11] necessitates evaporation of residual ether, and the digitonin-acid procedure of Jenkins and Moore[12] involves tedious washing of stroma. However, both methods can be undertaken within one hour. All other procedures can be performed within 30 minutes.

Hazards of Organic Solvents

Technologists may refrain from performing elution methods that utilize organic solvents in light of regulations imposed on the use of such reagents by federal agencies and safety authorities. These restrictions have been reviewed by Spivey.[96]

Organic solvents may be highly flammable (ether, flashpoint −49 F; xylene, flashpoint −81 F), and are considered carcinogenic (xylene, chloroform, DMSO). All four substances are toxic at high concentrations, and ether, chloroform and xylene can induce narcosis. Allergic reactions from skin contact have been reported with xylene and DMSO.[97] Consequently, care should be exercised when using these substances, and the necessary precautions (which are nothing more than common sense) followed. Bulk quantities of flammable organic solvents should be stored in an explosion-proof cabinet. However, small amounts (eg, four ounces) may be kept in opened canisters providing the contents are to be used within 30 days.[98] Organic solvents with flashpoints below 140 F should never be stored in a household refrigerator, where combustion triggered by electrical ignition sources might occur. Also, ether reacts with atmospheric oxygen to form peroxides, which are highly explosive. Since this reaction is catalyzed by light, ether should never be stored in clear glass containers. Both ether and xylene should be used in a well-ventilated area, away from heat, flame and sparks. Chloroform must be used in a well-ventilated area, preferably under a chemical hood.

Comparative Studies: Elution of Alloantibodies

Early Data

The earliest reported comprehensive study on the comparative sensitivity of various elution techniques is that of Jensen,[95] who evaluated the procedures described prior to 1957.[1,2,4-9] The methods of van

201

Loghem et al[6] and Weiner[9] were found to be superior to all other techniques for the elution of anti-A, anti-D, and warm-reactive auto-antibodies. Greenwalt's method[8] gave comparable results to the Landsteiner and Miller technique,[1] and both were considerably more sensitive than the remaining procedures.

Rubin[11] compared his ether technique with some of the earlier de-scribed elution techniques. Using red cells coated in vitro with anti-D, he found his method to compare favorably with that of Vos and Kel-sall.[5] Greenwalt's method[8] was the least sensitive, followed by the Landsteiner and Miller[1] and Weiner[9] procedures.

The only other major comparative study reported prior to 1970 is that undertaken by Hughes-Jones et al.[20] These investigators used ^{131}I-labeled anti-D to compare freeze-thaw, heat, ether, acid and alkali elution techniques. The original Rubin procedure,[11] which does not include incubation of the ether-red cell mixture at 37 C, was found to yield 50% of bound antibody. This increased to 70% when such incu-bation was undertaken for 30 minutes. In comparison, Weiner's technique[9] was the least sensitive (36% of bound antibody recovered), followed by heat at 56 C (43%), acid at pH 3.5 (80%) and alkali (87% at pH 11.3). However, antibody recovered in eluates at an alkaline pH was unstable; only 60% of eluted antibody was present in a serologi-cally active form. The authors attributed this observation to irreversi-ble changes to the tertiary structure of proteins caused by the alkaline environment.

Recent Studies by Original Authors

Table 2 presents a summary of comparative studies by those authors who have described new elution techniques within the past decade. While some reports include comparisons with some of the earlier de-scribed elution techniques, for the purpose of simplification, only data pertaining to the procedures included in the Appendices of this chapter and the AABB *Technical Manual*[43] have been tabulated. Also, Table 2 presents only the results of studies on red cells coated with alloantibodies in vitro.

This author will make no comment on the fact that all of the original authors claim superiority for their respective techniques; suffice it to say that the data do demonstrate such a bias. More importantly, it is clear that the heat elution technique is not the method of choice for eluting alloantibodies, as shown by the data of Jenkins and Moore[12] and Rekvig and Hannestad.[13] Perhaps of greater importance are the observations of Branch and Petz[19] and Bueno et al[18] that anti-s and anti-S antibodies are not readily eluted by ether.

202

Table 2.—Elution Methods: Comparative Studies on Red Cells Coated with IgG Alloantibodies in Vitro

Investigators	Comparative Effectiveness*	Antibody Specificity
Original Authors		
Jenkins and Moore[12]	DA > E > H	CD+Fy^a, D
	DA ≡ E, E > H	CD(2)
	E > DA > H	D
Rekvig and Hannestad[13]	CA > E > H	C, D
	CA > E, E ≡ H	K
	CA ≡ E ≡ H	Fy^a
Chan-Shu and Blair[17]	X > E	c, C, D, e, Fy^a, K
	X ≡ E	E
Bueno et al[18]	X > E	c(2), C, D(3), E(2), e
		Fy^a, Jk^a, Jr^a, k, K
		Yt^a
	X ≡ E	Fy^a(2), Fy^b, Jk^a, k(2)
		K(2), Kp^b(3), U
	X > DA, DA ≡ H, neg-E	Di^b, s(2), S(3)
	X > DA, neg-H, neg-E	E, Fy^b, S
Branch and Petz[19]	C ≡ X ≡ E	c, CD, D, E, Jk^a, Jk^b, s
	C ≡ X, neg-E	S
	C, neg-X, neg-E	S
	E ≡ X, X > C	Fy^a
Jimmerfield[24]	U > E > H	various (1912)
Independent Studies		
Ellisor et al[99]	†E > DA > H	E, k, K
	E > DA >> H	C, D, E, K
	E > DA, DA ≡ H	E, Jk^a, k
	E > DA, neg-H	D, Jk^a, K
	E ≡ DA, DA > H	D
	E ≡ DA ≡ H	Fy^a(2)
	E ≡ DA, neg-H	Fy^a, Jk^a, K
	E > H > DA	CD
	DA > E > H	K
	DA > E, E >> H	D
	DA >> E, neg-H	Fy^a
	DA, neg-E, neg-H	k

Table 2.—Elution Methods: Comparative Studies on Red Cells Coated with IgG Alloantibodies in Vitro—Cont.

Investigators	Comparative Effectiveness*	Antibody Specificity
Independent Studies—Cont.		
Gibble et al[100]	E > X > DA > CA > H	D
	E > DA	c, E
	DA > E	K
Reyes and S.M. Steane‡	X > E > DA	C
	X > E, E ≡ DA	s
	X ≡ E, E > DA	c, D(2), E, Fy^a
	X ≡ E ≡ DA	Fy^a, Fy^b, k, K(3)
	X ≡ E, neg-DA	c, Jk^a
	E > X, neg-DA	c, E, Jk^b
	E, neg-X, neg-DA	D

( ) Denotes number tested when more than one.
*C = chloroform; CA = cold acid; DA = digitonin-acid; E = ether; H = heat
U = ultrasound; X = xylene.
> = better than; ≡ = equivalent to; neg- = nonreactive.
†Ether elution plus 56 C heat.
‡Personal communication.

Studies by Independent Investigators

Also included in Table 2 are the results of comparative studies by independent investigators. Their findings conflict with those of the original investigators. The most comprehensive data reported are those of Ellisor,[99] who found a modified ether elution technique to be superior to digitonin-acid and heat for elution of most alloantibodies. Ether elution also performed favorably in the studies of Gibble et al,[100] and Reyes and S.M. Steane (personal communication). Of particular note, is the fact that some Kidd antibodies are not detectable in eluates prepared by the digitonin-acid technique.

In addition to the data summarized in Table 2, Ellisor et al[99] compared the Lui easy-freeze technique (Appendix 2) with that of heat elution. With few exceptions, the results were comparable, demonstrating that this freeze-thaw procedure also is not optimal for the elution of alloantibodies. Further, Cousins and Schanfield[101] compared digitonin-ether with digitonin-acid elution. Their findings support the contention that no single elution technique can be expected to detect all examples of alloantibodies.

Comparative Studies on Red Cells with a Positive DAT

It would appear that the majority of comparative studies have been performed on red cells coated with alloantibodies in vitro. Some reports do, however, include the results of a few tests on blood samples with a positive DAT. The results of all published data pertaining to the techniques included in the AABB *Technical Manual*[43] and in the Appendices of this chapter are summarized in Table 3. In addition, Table 3 includes the unpublished observations of Reyes and S.M. Steane, and those performed in this author's laboratory.

It is unfortunate that the report of Jimerfield[24] does not detail the grades of reactions with each sample studied, and his conclusions are based only on the combined data from all tests. We (Steiner EA, and Judd WJ, unpublished observations) concur that the sonication procedure is somewhat superior to heat for elution of anti-A and anti-B from cord blood samples. However, we found that sonication failed to elute anti-E from the red cells of an infant affected with Rh hemolytic disease. Further, we have found the cold-acid elution technique of Rekvig and Hannestad[13] to be ineffective for elution of transfusion-induced alloantibodies associated with in vivo sensitization of red cells.

While all of the data shown in Table 3 are somewhat limited, it is again noticeable that the results of the original investigators[12,13,17,18,24] support the superiority of their respective elution procedures. Such conclusions are conflicting, and are not supported by our own observations or those of Reyes and S.M. Steane (unpublished observations) and Ellisor et al.[99]

Comments on the Evaluation of Elution Techniques

Selection of Samples

It would seem inappropriate to use potent alloantibodies when sensitizing red cells in vitro for the purpose of evaluating elution techniques. Rather, due to the concentration effect of the adsorption-elution process, sera should be diluted to within one or two tubes below their titration endpoints to produce weakly sensitized cell samples. Further, while there is always the problem of obtaining sufficient quantities of blood, every attempt should be made to include samples from patients whose red cells are coated with auto- or alloantibodies in vivo. Such testing seems a more realistic approach to the evaluation of

Table 3.—Elution Methods: Comparative Studies on Blood Samples with a Positive DAT

| Investigators | Comparative Effectiveness* | Blood Samples Studied: | | | |
		Adult-Auto	Adult-Allo	Cord-ABO	Cord-Allo
Jenkins and Moore[12]	DA > E	7			
Rekvig and Hannestad[13]	CA > E > H	1			
	CA > E, E ≡ H			2	
Chan-Shu and Blair[17]	X > E	1	1(C)		
	X ≡ E	1			
	X, neg-E		1(C+Jk^b)		
Bueno et al[18]	X > E	9			
	X ≡ E	4			
	X > DA > H, neg-E	1			
	X, neg-E, neg-DA, neg-H	1		8	
	X > H			2	
	X ≡ H				

	181	799
Jimmerfield[24] — U > E > H		
Ellisor et al[99]		
E > DA, neg-H	1	
E ≡ DA, DA > H	1	
E ≡ DA, DA >> H	1	
E ≡ DA, neg-H	3	
DA > E, neg-H	2	
Reyes and S.M. Steane†		
E > X > DA	1	
E > X, X ≡ DA	1	
E > X, neg-DA	2	
E ≡ X ≡ DA	3(1 penicillin)	1(Jk^a)
E ≡ X, X > DA		1(U)
X ≡ DA		1(E)
		1(E)
Steiner and Judd†		
U > H		11
U ≡ H		7
H, neg-U		
E > CA	6	
E >> CA	3(E, cE, passive-A)	1(D)
E, neg-CA	2(Jk^a, E+Fy^a)	1(E)
	1(Jk^b)	

* CA = cold acid; E = ether; DA = digitonin acid; H = heat; X = xylene; U = ultrasound. > = better than; ≡ = equivalent to; neg- = nonreactive; ( ) denotes antibody specificity.
†Unpublished observations.

elution techniques, since it ensures the detection of eluted antibodies from "authentic" as opposed to artificially prepared samples.

Analysis of Eluates

With but one exception, all of the data summarized in Tables 2 and 3 are based on this author's interpretation of either titration score values or a difference of at least one grade in the degree of agglutination recorded in the various published and unpublished studies. Clearly, these interpretations are subjective, as are the test methods used by the authors concerned. For this reason, Gibble et al[100] used the enzyme-linked antiglobulin test (ELAT), as described by Leikola and Perkins,[102] to measure the amount of antibody recovered by elution. The use of radioiodinated antibodies as performed by Hughes-Jones et al,[20] or automated quantitative hemagglutination test systems, might eliminate errors due to the subjective reading of manual test reactions. However, while the precise measurement of eluted antibody by these methods might be advocated, this author does not wish to imply that manual test results are invalid. On the contrary, it can be argued that comparative studies on elution methods should be performed using only the routine techniques by which eluates are intended to be tested in the clinical situation.

Conclusions

A summary of the preceding discussion of the selection of elution techniques is given in Table 4. Until more detailed studies have been performed, the choice of a particular method for routine clinical use will remain one of personal preference based on convenience of use, with the stipulation that heat, freeze-thaw and sonication appear equally acceptable for studies in ABO hemolytic disease of the newborn, and techniques utilizing acid or organic solvents are necessary for optimal detection of warmreactive auto- and alloantibodies. It is difficult to draw further conclusions from the data shown in Tables 2 and 3 since the results of comparative studies are conflicting and in many instances only limited studies have been performed. In particular, it is apparent that ether eluates may fail to detect anti-S/s and digitonin-acid techniques may fail to detect anti-Kidd antibodies. However, it is evident that no single elution technique will suffice for the detection of all antibodies. Thus, when unexpected negative elution studies are encountered, several different procedures should be applied. This is obviously important when evaluating blood samples from patients manifesting clinical symptoms of an immune response to recently transfused red cells.

Table 4.—Elution Methods; Advantages and Disadvantages

Method	Time Required*	Advantages	Disadvantages
Heat	15 min.	Quick; good for ABO HDN	Poor sensitivity for warm auto- and alloantibodies
Ether	50 min.	Good sensitivity for most warm auto- and alloantibodies	Highly flammable; narcotic; toxic; tedious evaporation of ether insensitive for anti-S/s
Digitonin-Acid	35 min.	Nonhazardous	Tedious washing of stroma; less sensitive than ether; insensitive for some alloantibodies (especially Kidd)
Cold Acid	10 min.	Quick	Dubious sensitivity for warm auto- and alloantibodies
Freeze-Thaw	15 min.	Quick; good for ABO HDN	Poor sensitivity for warm auto- and alloantibodies
Xylene	25 min.	Less flammable than ether	Flammable; carcinogenic; narcotic; toxic
Chloroform	20 min.	Nonflammable	Carcinogenic; narcotic; toxic
Sonication	5 min.	Quick; good for ABO HDN	Dubious sensitivity for warm auto- and alloantibodies

* Excluding time required to wash the red cells prior to elution.

Acknowledgments

I would like to thank Virginia Reyes and Susan Steane (Parkland Memorial Hospital Blood Bank, Dallas, TX), and Sandra Ellisor (American Red Cross Blood Program, San Jose, CA) for permission to include their comparative data in Tables 2 and 3. I am indebted to Kim Drake for secretarial assistance, and to M. Jane Wilson, Dr. Edwin Steane, and my colleagues at the University of Michigan for their invaluable comments and constructive criticism of this manuscript.

Appendix 1

Cold Acid Elution
(Method of Rekvig and Hannestad[13])

Materials

0.1 M glycine: prepared by dissolving 3.754 g of glycine and 2.922 g of sodium chloride in 500 ml of distilled water. Adjust pH to 3.0 with 12 N HCl. Store at 4 C.

0.8 M phosphate buffer at pH 8.2: prepared by dissolving 109.6 g of Na_2HPO_4 and 3.8 g of KH_2PO_4 in approximately 600 ml of distilled water and adjust pH to 8.2 (if necessary) with either 1 N NaOH or 1 N HCL.

Packed red cells (1 ml): washed six times in saline (save final wash supernatant).

Isotonic saline: chilled to 4 C.

Method

1. To 1 ml of washed packed red cells in a 13 x 100 mm test tube, add 1 ml of chilled saline and 2 ml of glycine (see note #1).
2. Mix, and incubate the tube in an ice bath for one minute.
3. Centrifuge the tube at 1,000 x g for two minutes.
4. Transfer the supernatant eluate into a clean test tube and add 0.1 ml of pH 8.2 phosphate buffer for each 1 ml of eluate (see note #2).
5. Mix, and centrifuge the tube at 1,000 x g for two minutes.
6. Transfer the supernatant eluate into a clean test tube, and test in parallel with the final wash supernatant.

Notes

1. Keep glycine at 4 C during use.
2. Phosphate buffer will crystallize on storage at 4 C. Redissolve at 37 C prior to use.

Appendix 2

Lui Easy-Freeze Elution
(After Barnes[16])

Materials

Packed red cells: washed six times in saline (save final wash supernatant).

Method

1. Dispense 0.5 ml of washed packed red cells into a 13 x 100 mm test tube (prepare sufficient tubes to yield the amount of eluate required).
2. Add three drops of saline to each tube of red cells and mix well.
3. Stopper the tubes, and rotate them so as to coat the inside surface of the tubes with red cells.
4. Place the tubes horizontally at between −20 C and −70 C for ten minutes.
5. Rapidly thaw the red cells under running warm tap water.
6. Centrifuge the tubes at 1,000 x g for two minutes.
7. Transfer the supernatant eluate into a clean test tube, and test in parallel with the final wash supernatant.

Appendix 3

Xylene Elution[18]

Materials

Xylene: reagent grade (Mallinckrodt Inc.)
Packed red cells (2 ml): washed six times in saline (save final wash supernatant).

Method

1. Mix equal volumes of washed packed red cells and xylene in a 13 x 100 mm test tube.
2. Stopper the tube, and agitate it vigorously for one to two minutes.
3. Place the tube at 56 C for ten minutes, agitating it periodically during this time.
4. Centrifuge the tube at 1,000 x g for ten minutes.
5. Carefully remove the upper layer of xylene and the stroma by vacuum aspiration (see note #1).
6. Transfer the eluate into a clean test tube and test in parallel with the final wash supernatant.

Notes

1. Care should be taken not to contaminate the eluate with stroma (avoid using a Pasteur pipette to remove xylene and stroma). If contamination of eluate does occur, recentrifuge at 1,000 x g for 10 minutes to remove particulate matter.
2. This procedure is a modification of the method described by Chan-Shu and Blair.[17]

Appendix 4

Chloroform Elution
(After Branch et al[17])

Materials

Chloroform: reagent grade (Mallinkrodt Inc.).
6% bovine albumin: diluted from stock 22% or 30% bovine albumin with saline.
Packed red cells (1 ml): washed six times in saline (save final wash supernatant).

Method

1. To 1 ml of washed packed red cells in a 13 x 100 mm test tube add 1 ml of 6% albumin and two ml of chloroform.
2. Stopper the tube with a cork, and agitate the tube vigorously for 15 seconds. Mix further by inversion for one minute.
3. Remove the cork, and place the tube at 56 C for five minutes. Stir the contents of the tube with an applicator stick during this time.

4. Centrifuge the tube at 1,000 x g for five minutes.
5. Transfer the eluate (upper layer) into a clean test tube and test in parallel with the final wash supernatant.

Appendix 5

Elution by Sonication[24]

Materials

Ultrasound cleaning bath: American Scientific Products
6% bovine albumin: prepared from stock 22% or 30% bovine albumin by dilution with saline.
Packed red cells (2 ml): washed six times in saline (save final wash supernatant).

Method

1. Mix one volume of 6% bovine albumin and two volumes of washed packed red cells in a 13 x 100 mm test tube.
2. Fill the ultrasound cleaning bath to within one inch of the top with distilled water, and switch on.
3. Place the tube in the center of the water bath, resting the bottom of the tube on the bottom of the water bath.
4. Maintain the tube in this position for approximately one minute (until lysis of the red cells is complete). Mixing the contents of the tube with a Pasteur pipette will reduce the time needed for complete hemolysis.
5. Centrifuge the tube at 1,000 x g for five minutes.
6. Transfer the supernatant eluate into a clean test tube, and test in parallel with the final wash supernatant.

Appendix 6

Chloroquine Dissociation of IgG
(After Edwards et al[28])

Materials

Chloroquine diphosphate: 20% (w/v) in saline. Adjust pH to 5.1 with 5 N NaOH.
Packed red cells (IgG-coated): washed three times in saline.

Anti-IgG reagent: monospecific or oligospecific (devoid of anticomplement components) anti-IgG.

Method

1. To 0.2 ml of washed packed red cells add 0.8 ml of chloroquine diphosphate solution.
2. Mix, and incubate at room temperature for 30 minutes.
3. Remove a small aliquot of the chloroquine-treated red cells and wash four times in saline.
4. To one drop of a 5% saline suspension of these washed red cells, add anti-IgG according to the manufacturer's directions.
5. Centrifuge at 1,000 x g for 15 seconds.
6. Examine the red cells macroscopically for agglutination:

if nonreactive: wash all of the chloroquine-treated red cells and use for phenotyping with antisera that require use by the indirect antiglobulin technique. Use an anti-IgG reagent for such testing.

if reactive: repeat steps 3-5 at 30 minute intervals, until the red cells are nonreactive with anti-IgG. Then use for phenotyping as described above.

Note

Edwards et al[28] used chloroquine diphosphate from Sterling Organics, Northumberland, England. A slightly different, and less effective, formulation is obtainable from Sigma Chemical Company, St. Louis, MO.

References

1. Landsteiner K, Miller CP Jr. Serological studies on the blood of primates. II. The blood groups in anthropoid apes. J. Exp Med 1925;42:853-62.
2. Kidd P. Elution of an incomplete type of antibody from the erythrocytes in acquired haemolytic anaemia. J Clin Pathol 1949; 2:103-8.
3. Landsteiner K, van der Scheer J. On cross reactions of immune sera to azoproteins. J Exp Med 1936;63:325-39.
4. Komninos ZD, Rosenthal MC. Studies on antibodies eluted from the red cells in autoimmune hemolytic anemia. J Lab Clin Med 1953;41:887-94.

5. Vos GH, Kelsall GA. A new elution technique for the preparation of specific immune anti-Rh serum. Br J Haematol 1956;2:342-4.

6. van Loghen JJ, Mendes de Leon DE, van der Hart M. Recherches serologiques dans les anemies hemolytiques acquises. 30th Congr Franc Med, Alger, 1955. Paris: Masson, 1957.

7. Selwyn JG. Doctoral thesis, Cambridge University, 1952. Cited in: Dacie JV. The acquired haemolytic anaemias—congenital and acquired. London: Churchill, 1954:494-5.

8. Greenwalt TJ. A method for eluting antibodies from red cell stromata. J Lab Clin Med 1956;48:634-6.

9. Weiner W. Eluting red-cell antibodies: a method and its application. Brit J Haematol 1957;3:276-83.

10. Kochwa S, Rosenfield RE. Immunochemical studies of the Rh system. I. Isolation and characterization of antibodies. J Immunol 1964;92:682-92.

11. Rubin H. Antibody elution from red blood cells. J Clin Pathol 1963;16:70-3.

12. Jenkins DE, Moore WH. A rapid method for the preparation of high-potency auto and alloantibody eluates. Transfusion 1977; 17:110-4.

13. Rekvig OP, Hannestad K. Acid elution of blood group antibodies from intact erythrocytes. Vox Sang 1977;33:280-5.

14. Bush M. A modified one-stage acid elution technique for allo- and autoantibodies, abstract. Transfusion 1978;18:388.

15. Eicher CA, Wallace ME, Frank S, de Jongh DS. The Lui elution: a simple freezing method for antibody elution, abstract. Transfusion 1978;18:647.

16. Barnes JM. Evaluation of the Lui easy freeze elution test. Lab Med 1981;12:227-8.

17. Chan-Shu SA, Blair O. A new method of antibody elution from red blood cells. Transfusion 1979;19:182-5.

18. Bueno R, Garratty G, Postoway N. Elution of antibody from red blood cells using xylene—a superior method. Transfusion 1981; 21:157-62.

19. Branch DR, Sy Siok Hian AL, Petz LD. A new elution procedure using a nonflammable organic solvent, abstract. Transfusion 1980;20:635.

20. Hughes-Jones NC, Gardner B, Telford R. Comparison of various methods of dissociation of anti-D, using ^{131}I-labelled antibody. Vox Sang 1963;8:531-6.

21. Edgington TS. Dissociation of antibody from erythrocyte surfaces by chaotropic ions. J Immunol 1971;106:673-80.

22. van Oss CJ, Beckers D, Engelfriet CP, Absolom DR, Neumann AW. Elution of blood group antibodies from red cells. Vox Sang 1981;40:367-71.

23. Bird GWG, Wingham J. A new method for elution of erythrocyte-bound antibody. Acta Haematol 1972;47:344-7.

24. Jimerfield CA. A rapid and simple method for preparing red cell eluates using ultrasound. J Amer Med Technol 1977;39:187-9.

25. Mantel W, Holtz G. Characterisation of autoantibodies to erythrocytes in autoimmune haemolytic anaemia by chloroquine. Vox Sang 1976;30:453-63.

26. Holtz G, Mantel W, Buck W. The inhibition of antigen-antibody reactions by chloroquine and its mechanism of action. Z Immun-Forsch 1973;146:145-57.

27. Mantel W, Holtz G. The inhibition of antigen-antibody reaction by quinoline derivatives. Z Immun-Forsch 1974;147:420-30.

28. Edwards JM, Moulds JJ, Judd WJ. Chloroquine diphosphate: a new technique for phenotyping red cells having a positive direct antiglobulin test Transfusion 1982;22:59-61.

29. Howard PL. Principles of antibody elution. Transfusion 1981;21:477-83.

30. van Oss CJ, Grossberg AL. Antigen-antibody interactions. In: Principles of immunology. 2nd ed. Rose NR, Milgrom F, van Oss CJ, eds. New York: Macmillan, 1979:65-79.

31. Calvin M, Evans RS, Behrendt V, Calvin G. Rh antigen and hapten: nature of antigen and its isolation from erythrocyte stroma. Proc Soc Exp Biol Med 1946;61:416-9.

32. Lubinski HH, Portnuff JC. The influence of heat and formalin on the Rh agglutinogen. J Lab Clin Med 1947;32:178-80.

33. Hubinont PO. Action of heating on Rh-positive human red cells. Nature 1948;161:642.

34. Ballas SK, Miguel O. Effect of temperature on the red cell membrane protein and its antigenic reactivity. Transfusion 1981;21:537-41.

35. Hurn BAL. Storage of blood. London: Academic Press, 1968:50-7.

36. Muller CP, Shinitzky M. Passive shedding of erythrocyte antigens induced by membrane rigidification. Exp Cell Res 1981;136:53-62.

37. Steane EA. The interaction of antibodies with red cell surface antigens: kinetics, noncovalent bonding, and hemagglutination. In: Blood bank immunology. Washington DC: American Association of Blood Banks, 1977:61-85.

38. Dandliker WH, Alonso JR, de Saussure VA, Kierszenbaum S, Levison SA, Schapiro HC. The effect of chaotropic ions on the dissociation of antigen antibody complexes. Biochemistry 1967;6: 1460-7.

39. Ruoslathi E. Antigen-antibody interaction, antibody affinity, and dissociation of immune complexes. Scand J Immunol 1976;3: 3-5.

40. van Oss CJ, Absolom DR, Neumann AW. The "hydrophobic effect": essentially a van der Waals interaction. Colloid and Polymer Sci 1980;258:424-7.

41. Hughes-Jones NC, Gardner B, Telford R. Studies on the reaction between the blood-group antibody anti-D and erythrocytes. Biochem J 1963;88:435-40.

42. van Oss CJ, Absolom DR, Neumann AW. Applications of net repulsive van der Waals forces between different particles, macromolecules or biological cells in liquids. Colloids and surfaces 1980;1:45-56.

43. Technical manual. 8th ed. Washington DC: American Association of Blood Banks, 1981.

44. Matuhasi T. Plasma protein and antibody fractions observed from the serological point of view. Proc 15th General Assembly Jap Med Congr, Tokyo 1959;4:80-7.

45. Matuhasi T, Kumazawa H, Usui M. Question of the presence of so-called cross-reacting antibody. J Jap Soc Blood Transf 1960;6: 295-7.

46. Allen FH Jr., Issitt PD, Degnan TJ, et al. Further observations on the Mathuhasi-Ogata phenomenon. Vox Sang 1969;16:47-56.

47. Ogata T, Matuhasi T. Problems of specific and cross reactivity of blood group antibodies. Proc 8th Congr Int Soc Blood Transf, 1960. Basel: Karger 1962:208-11.

48. Ogata T, Matuhasi T. Further observations on the problems of specific and cross reactivity blood group antibodies. Proc 9th Congr Int Soc Blood Transf, 1962. Basel: Karger 1964:528-31.

49. Svardal JM, Yarbro J, Yunis EJ. Ogata phenomenon explaining the unusual specificity in eluates from Coombs positive cells sensitized by autogenous anti-I. Vox Sang 1967;13:472-84.

50. Dunsford I, Stapleton RR. In vitro absorption of the rhesus antibody anti-D by rhesus negative red cells. Vox Sang 1959;4:406-8.

51. Boursnell JC, Coombs RRA, Rizk V. Studies with marked antisera: quantitative studies with antisera marked with iodine [131]isotope and their corresponding red-cell antigens. Biochem J 1953;55:745-58.

52. Pirofsky B, Cordova MS, Imel TI. The nonimmunologic reaction of globulin molecules with the erythrocyte surface. Vox Sang 1962;7:334-47.

53. Gergely J, Medgyesi GA, Horvath E. Specific binding of γG globulin to erythrocytes. Vox San 1966;11:724-5.

54. Gergely J, Arky I, Medgyesi GA. Nonspecific interaction of the papain insensitive and papain sensitive populations of human IgG with erythrocytes. Vox Sang 1967;12:252-64.

55. Bove JR, Holburn AM, Mollison PL. Non-specific binding of IgG to antibody-coated red cells (the 'Matuhasi-Ogata phenomenon'). Immunology 1973;25:793-801.

56. McKeever BG. Further observations on the Matuhasi-Ogata Phenomenon, MS thesis. University of Cincinnati, 1974.

57. Wilkinson SL, Vaithianathan T, Issitt PD. The high incidence of anti-HLA antibodies in anti-D typing reagents. Illustrated by a case of Matuhasi-Ogata phenomenon mimicking a "D with anti-D" situation. Transfusion 1974;14:27-33.

58. Issitt PD, Issitt CH. Applied blood group serology. 2nd ed. Oxnard: Spectra Biologicals, 1975.

59. Issitt PD, Pavone BG, Wagstaff W, Goldfinger D. The phenotypes En(a−), Wr(a−b−) and En(a+), Wr(a+b−), and further studies on the Wright and En[a] blood group systems. Transfusion 1976;16: 396-407.

60. Masouredis SP, Mahan LC, Sudora EJ, Langley JW, Victoria EJ. Estimation of anti-D IgG in red blood cell eluates using the specific radioactivity of ^{125}I-labeled IgG: effect of unlabeled, cytophilic IgG. Transfusion 1981;21:377-83.

61. Case J, Moulds JJ. On rh[G] (C[G]) and related matters, letter. Transfusion 1982;22:258-259.

62. Mollison PL. Blood transfusion in clinical medicine. 6th ed. Oxford: Blackwell Scientific Publications, 1979.

63. Judd WJ, Jenkins WJ. Automated antibody (anti-D) quantitation technique, letter. J Clin Pathol 1972;25:916.

64. Voak D, Williams MA. An explanation of the failure of the direct antiglobulin test to detect erythrocyte sensitization in ABO haemolytic disease of the newborn and observations on pinocytosis of IgG anti-A antibodies by infant (cord) red cells. Br J Haematol 1971;20:9-23.

65. Romano EL, Hughes-Jones NC, Mollison PL. Direct antiglobulin reactions in ABO hemolytic disease of the newborn. Br Med J 1973;i:524.

66. Petz LD, Garratty G. Acquired immune hemolytic anemias. New York: Churchill Livingstone, 1980.
67. Romans DG, Tilley CA, Dorrington KJ. Monogamous bivalency of IgG antibodies. I. Deficiency of branched ABHI-active oligosaccharide chains on red cells of infants causes the weak antiglobulin reaction in hemolytic disease of the newborn due to ABO incompatibility. J Immunol 1980;124:2807-11.
68. Clinical aspects of the positive direct antiglobulin test. Washington, DC: American Association of Blood Banks, 1980.
69. A seminar on immune mediated red cell destruction. Washington, DC: American Association of Blood Banks, 1981.
70. Issitt PD. Autoimmune hemolytic anemia and cold hemagglutinin disease: clinical disease and laboratory findings. Progr Clin Pathol 1977;7:137-63.
71. Pirofsky B. Autoimmunization and the autoimmune hemolytic anemias. Baltimore: Williams and Wilkins, 1969.
72. Garratty G. Drug-related problems. In: A seminar on problems encountered in pretransfusion tests. Washington, DC: American Association of Blood Banks, 1972:33-58.
73. Hollander L. Study of erythrocyte survival time in a case of acquired haemolytic anaemia. Vox Sang (O.S.) 1954;4:164-8.
74. Judd WJ, Butch SH, Oberman HA, Steiner EA, Bauer RC. The evaluation of a positive direct antiglobulin test in pretransfusion testing. Transfusion 1980;20:17-23.
75. Worlledge SM. The interpretation of a positive direct antiglobulin test, annotation. Br J Haematol 1978;39:157-62.
76. Freedman J. False positive antiglobulin tests in healthy subjects and in hospital patients. J Clin Pathol 1979;32:1014-8.
77. Fudenberg HH, Rosenfield RE, Wasserman LR. Unusual specificity of autoantibody in auto-immune hemolytic anemia. J Mt Sinai Hosp 1958;25:324-9.
78. Issitt PD, Zellner DC, Rolih SD, Duckett JB. Autoantibodies mimicking alloantibodies. Transfusion 1977;17:531-8.
79. Issitt PD, Pavone BG, Shapiro M. Anti-Rh 39: a "new" specificity Rh system antibody. Transfusion 1979;19:389-97.
80. Hare V, Wilson MJ, Wilkinson S, Issitt PD. A Kell system antibody with highly unusual characteristics, abstract. Transfusion 1981;21:613.
81. Levine P, Uhlir M, White J. A_h, an incomplete suppression of A resembling O_h. Vox Sang 1961;6:561-7.
82. Stanbury A, Francis B. The Lu(a−b−) phenotype: an additional example. Vox Sang 1967;13:441-3.

83. Vos G. The evaluation of specific anti-G (CD) eluate obtained by a double adsorption and elution procedure. Vox Sang 1960;5: 472-8.

84. van der Hart M, Szaloky A, van Loghem JJ. A 'new' antibody in the Kell blood group system. Vox Sang 1968;15:456-8.

85. Issitt PD. MN blood group system. Cincinnati: Montgomery Scientific, 1981.

86. Marsh WL. Scoring of hemagglutination reactions. Transfusion 1972;12:352-3.

87. Beattie KM. Laboratory investigation and management of antibody specificities in warm autoimmune hemolytic anemia. In: A seminar on laboratory management of hemolysis. Washington, DC: American Association of Blood Banks, 1979:105-34.

88. Goldstein IJ, Hayes CE. The lectins: carbohydrate-binding proteins of plants and animals. Adv Carbohyd Chem Biochem 1978;35:127-340.

89. Anstee DJ, Barker DM, Judson PA, Tanner MJA. Inherited sialoglycoprotein deficiencies in human erythrocytes of type En(a−). Br J Haematol 1977;35:309-20.

90. Reid ME. Autoagglutination dispersal utilizing sulphydryl compounds. Transfusion 1978;18:353-5.

91. Branch DR, Petz LD. A new reagent having multiple applications in immunohematology, abstract. Transfusion 1980;20:642.

92. Morel PA, Bergren MO, Frank BA. A simple method for the detection of alloantibody in the presence of autoantibody, abstract. Transfusion 1978;18:388.

93. Moulds J, Mallory D, Zodin V. Placental eluates: an economical source of antibodies, abstract. Transfusion 1978;18:388.

94. Lincoln PJ, Dodd BE. The application of a micro-elution technique using anti-human globulin for the detection of the S, s, K, Fy^a, Fy^b and Jk^a antigens in stains. Med Sci Law 1975;15:94-101.

95. Jensen KG. Elution of incomplete antibody from red cells: a comparison of different methods. Vox Sang 1959;4:230-9.

96. Spivey MA. Laboratory safety in relation to chemical elution techniques. Red Cell Free Press 1981;6:10.

97. The Merck Index, 9th ed. Rahway, NJ: Merck, 1976.

98. National Safety Council. Flammable and combustible liquids. Occupational Safety and Health Administration Standards. Washington DC, 1972; Subpart H: Section 1910.106.

99. Ellisor SS, Reid ME, Marks M. Comparison of five elution procedures, abstract. Transfusion 1970;19:654.

100. Gibble JW, Salamon JL, Ness PM. Comparison of antibody elution techniques by enzyme-linked antiglobulin test (ELAT), abstract. Transfusion 1981;21:627.

101. Cousins CR, Schanfield MS. Variation in the susceptibility of different blood group antigens to elution: digitonin ether vs. acid, abstract. Transfusion 1978;18:631.

102. Leikola J, Perkins HA. Enzyme-linked antiglobulin test: an accurate and simple method to quantify red cell antibodies. Transfusion 1980;20:138-44.

9

The Use of Antigen-Antibody Techniques in Forensic Serology

Barbara E. Dodd, DSc, and Patrick J. Lincoln, PhD

Introduction

ANTIGEN-ANTIBODY PHENOMENA are well seen in operation in the detection of antigens in blood stains.

Before discussing the techniques used in this field, the situation facing the blood stain analyst must be appreciated. While the blood transfusion serologist tests a red cell suspension, the forensic serologist has to make do with a blood stained thread pulled, for example, from the coat of a suspected person. The blood transfusion serologist almost always has a more than adequate sample for testing, for although in some crimes blood staining is copious, in others only a trace amount of scarcely visible blood may be found on clothing or at the crime scene. Furthermore, the task of grouping stains is made harder because a blood stain does not yield intact red cells and may have been subjected to adverse conditions such as exposure to weather, contamination with other substances or the passage of time, before the opportunity to test it in the laboratory arrives.

Such are the constraints upon typing blood stains but in spite of them, research over the past 20 years or so has resulted in almost all the well-known red cell antigen systems and other polymorphisms, such as red cell enzymes and serum groups, being detectable in stains by using special modifications of well-known techniques. Since, however, this chapter forms part of a work devoted to antigen-antibody reaction, the authors shall confine their remarks to those genetic markers which are detectable in stains by methods which rely upon antigen-antibody principles.

Barbara E. Dodd, DSc, Professor of Blood Group Serology; and Patrick J. Lincoln, PhD, Senior Lecturer in Blood Group Serology, The London Hospital Medical College, London, England

The Typical Problem

The purpose of typing blood stains is, as far as possible, to identify their origin, whether from victim, suspect or other persons who may be associated with a crime. A blood stain may be excluded from originating from a given source with certainty, but positive proof of its origin inevitably rests on probability. Using the selected systems shown in Table 1, the expected success in making a distinction between two bloods having different sources is good.

Table 1.—The Expected Success in Distinguishing Between Bloods of Different Origin*

System	Expected % Success in Making Distinction on:	
	Individual Systems	Combined Systems
ABO (A,B,H)	67.2	
Rh (C,c,D,E,e)	80.5	
MNSs (MNSs)	83.6	98.9
Duffy (Fy^a, Fy^b)	63.3	
Kidd (Jk^a)	36.0	
Kell (K)	16.3	99.8
Gm (1,2)	64.7	
Km (1)	29.0	99.9

*Data from Lincoln.[1]

In practice, for various reasons, tests for the complete range of systems detectable on stain material are not made. In a typical case where a blood stain may be on a suspect's clothing, the results of a detailed blood group investigation of whole samples from both victim and suspect determines which antigens will be most useful to look for in the stain.[1] A system in which victim and suspect belong to different groups will almost certainly be investigated because results from such tests will indicate whether or not blood on the suspect's clothing can be his own or the victim's. Choices are also influenced by the size of the stain and its age. Red cell antigens are usually more resistant to the passage of time than are red cell enzyme markers. Antigen frequency is important, those antigens which are least common being preferentially selected. For example, the presence of C^w in either victim or suspect would be a godsend! However, even without finding uncommon phenotypes, valuable information may be obtained provided several systems are included.

Table 2 compares the grouping of whole blood from a victim with blood stains found on two areas of a pair of jeans belonging to his alleged assailant. One stain from the thigh area matches the blood group profile of the victim in all four systems investigated. This blood group combination occurs in only 0.1% of West Europeans. Test for PGM1 had to be omitted from the smaller stain on the pocket but even with this omission the frequency of the blood group combination is no higher than 3%. Blood stain evidence such as this taken within the context of the particular case has great evidential value.

Table 2.—The Value of Testing Stains for Several Systems*

	ABO	Rh D C E c	S	PGM1	Phenotype Frequency%
Blood group profile of victim	A	++++	+	2+	0.1
Blood stains from jeans:					
Thigh area	A	++++	+	2+	0.1
Pocket	A	++++	+		3.0

*Data from case work.

It is not even always necessary to test for more than a single system in order to gain important objective evidence. Table 3 records such an example. In this case, one man accused another of assaulting and wounding him using a milk crate as a weapon. However, the accused alleged that he was the one attacked and that he used the milk crate merely to protect himself from being injured by the alleged victim and also his wife.[2] There was light blood staining on the edge of the milk crate which the accused insisted was his own blood. Tests on the three people involved showed them each to have a different ABO group so after removing some of the stain onto cotton threads its ABO group was established as group B, thus supporting the statement of the accused, who was subsequently acquitted.

Table 3.—The Milk Crate Case*

	ABO Group
Accused person	B
Victim of alleged assault	A
Wife of victim	O
Blood stain on crate	B

*Data from Lincoln.[2]

The Principles of Inhibition, Mixed Agglutination and Elution as Applied to the Detection of Antigens in Blood Stains

A colleague once suggested that these three processes were analogous to dipping a mop (cellular antigen or blood stain) into a puddle (antiserum). Inhibition examines the puddle for what it may have lost, mixed agglutination investigates the mop itself or the mop may be squeezed (which constitutes elution).

Mixed Agglutination as a Method for the Detection of Antigen in Stains

The application of the mixed cell agglutination principle to the detection of antigens in stains will be briefly considered, for though it was heralded with acclaim when introduced by Coombs and Dodd,[3] it was found in practice to have limited application and was soon abandoned in favour of elution.

The principle of mixed agglutination was first applied by Coombs et al[4] as a method for detecting antigen in cells unsuited to direct agglutination techniques. The test cells, or in the case of blood stains, stained threads, are mixed with a suitable antiserum, eg, anti-A, and time is allowed for the combination of the antibody with the corresponding antigen in the stain. The threads are then washed to remove uncombined antibody and fresh red cells are added as indicator cells. These are chosen to possess the antigen under study, eg, antigen A. If the selected antiserum contains an agglutinating anti-A (preferably IgM), it initiates a mixed agglutination reaction, with the indicator cells becoming bound to the stained thread by the anti-A which is already specifically taken up by the A antigen of the stain but has free receptors available for the antigen of the indicator cells. A typical

226

positive is shown in Fig 1. The indicator cells usually align themselves in neat rows as seen here but occasionally they compete more successfully than the stain antigen for the available antibody, in which case a field of agglutinated cells is seen, in which the agglutinates do not remain attached to the stain. The technique is elegant but it was found that only a relatively small number of antisera were suitable for it, and it did not work satisfactorily for antigens of systems other than ABO. It has been superseded by a technique using the elution principle.

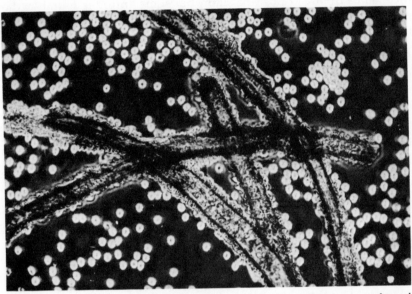

Fig 1.—A typical mixed agglutination appearance when the technique is performed using bloodstained threads. (Reproduced from Coombs & Dodd.[3])

The Micro-elution Technique for Antigens in Blood Stains

Over the years, an elution procedure based on the familiar Landsteiner heat elution technique has been developed.[5-7] The technique is "micro" in the sense that to be useful it has to be an adaptation of the heat elution procedure suited to very small amounts of antigen, ie, the quantity which remains active on one or two blood stained threads. The details of the technique for those who wish to use it are appended to this chapter. This section discusses points of interest relating to the three stages of the technique and includes the results of experiments designed to evaluate the factors affecting the elution of antibodies from blood stains.

The Absorption Stage

At this stage, the relative concentrations of antigen and antibody are important. For example, in adding a selected antiserum to a blood stained thread it is very easy to slip into the region of antibody excess. At best, this is unnecessary and at worst may lead to false positives due to the difficulty of washing away all traces of uncombined antibody as the experiments recorded in Table 4 illustrate. At lower dilutions than 1 in 100 there is no marked increase in yield of antibody recovered in the eluates from a D-positive stain, but some anti-D is found in the eluates made from a D-negative stain. Thus, the optimum dilution of this anti-D for typing stains is at least 1/100.

Table 4.—Elution from Decreasing Concentrations of Anti-D*

Anti-D Used For Absorption		Papain Titre of Eluates From	
Dilution:	Papain Titre	DccEE Stain	ddccee Stain
1/2	32,000	128	32
1/10	8,000	256	2
1/40	1,000	256	2
1/100	512	128	0
1/640	64	32	0

*Data from Lincoln & Dodd.[8]

It is also possible to overdo the antigen concentration. Table 5 shows the decreased yield of eluted anti-A when it is combined with more than the optimal amount of bloodstain.

Table 5.—The Effect on the Yield of Antibody of Decreasing the Amount of Bloodstain*

Titre of Anti-A Used for Absorption	Packed Cells Used as Bloodstains (ml)	Titre of Eluate
1,000	0.005	8
	0.0025	128
	0.00025	128

*Data from Lincoln & Dodd.[8]

The absorption may take place in tubes but for large scale work polycarbonate sheets are time savers. The tip of each stained thread is attached to the sheet using a cellulose acetate glue and the thread is then covered with two drops of antiserum. The period for which the stained threads and the appropriate antiserum remain in contact is usually overnight at the temperature most appropriate for the antigens under investigation.

After the absorption period, the sheets with attached threads are placed in a tank of ice-cold saline. At this temperature, there is minimum dissociation of any specifically bound antibody. After washing for two hours, the threads are transferred to tubes and one drop of 0.3% bovine albumin in PBS is added as elution fluid.

Elution Stage

Elution takes place over a period of 15 to 30 minutes in a shaking water bath at a temperature appropriate to the antibody being eluted. Table 6 shows the effect of varying the elution temperature on elution from blood stains of anti-A and anti-D. It is seen that the optimum temperature for anti-A is 55 C whereas elution of anti-D is optimal at 65 C. The difference is likely to be due to the fact that the anti-A is largely IgM and is therefore more heat labile than the IgG anti-D. Ideally, the optimum temperature for elution should be predetermined for each antibody selected for routine use. An elution period of 30 minutes is longer than is normal for this elution technique but it has been found that the longer time improves the antibody yield. Moreover, stained threads do not undergo haemolysis as do fresh red

Table 6.—Elution from Bloodstains of Anti-A and Anti-D at Various Temperatures*

	Titre of Eluates	
Elution Temp.	Anti-A Saline	Anti-D Papain
4 C	2	0
22 C	4	0
37 C	4	2
55 C	16	16
60 C	8	32
65 C	4	64

*Data from Lincoln & Dodd.[8]

cells when subjected to relatively high temperatures for a considerable period of time.

The next stage of the test is peculiar to elution of antibody from stained threads in that, instead of rapidly separating the eluted antibody from the antigen, fresh indicator red cells are added directly to the eluate without first removing the stained thread. Such a maneuver is not possible when eluting from red cells, but experience has shown that stronger agglutination of the indicator cells is obtained in the presence of the bloodstain than is obtained if the eluate is separated from the stain before the addition of the indicator cells. It appears that the indicator cells continue to acquire antibody both by competing successfully for any antibody remaining in dynamic equilibrium with the antigen of the stain and by combining with an antibody which, it is known, continues to elute from the stain.

Detection of Eluted Antibody

Since the eluted antibody originates from the very small amount of antigen present on a single stained thread of about 5 mm in length, its concentration in the eluate is very small and in order to achieve maximum sensitivity for its detection the antigen concentration of the indicator cells must be less than the normal concentration used for antibody detection tests (Table 7). The marked effect of the dilute

Table 7.—The Effect of Different Concentrations of Cell Suspensions for the Titration of Antibodies*

Dilution of Anti-c	% Concentration of Cell Suspension	Titre with Papain-Treated Cells
1/16	2	128
	0.5	512
	0.1	512
	0.05	512
1/64	2	32
	0.5	256
	0.1	256
	0.05	256
1/256	2	8
	0.5	32
	0.1	64
	0.05	128

*Data from Lincoln & Dodd.[8]

suspensions on the lowest concentration of antibody should be particularly noted.

A 0.1% suspension of papain-treated cells is used for all Rh antibodies. Experience has shown that a papain technique is considerably superior to antiglobulin for the detection of eluted Rh antibodies (Table 8). A 0.5% suspension of untreated cells is suitable for the detection of anti-A, anti-B or anti-H.

Table 8.—A Comparison Between Papain and AHG Techniques for the Titration of Eluted Anti-D*

Technique	Titre of Eluates Made at Various Temp (C)		
	50	55	60
Enzyme (papain)	128	1000	512
AHG	2	8	16

*Data from Lincoln & Dodd.[10]

When testing for the presence of antigens which require an antiglobulin technique (eg, S, s, Fy[a], Jk[a], etc.) a drop of 1% cells is added to each test without removing the stain, after which the tests are incubated for 1 hour at 37 C, the threads removed and an AHG test performed. In all cases, if a titration of the eluted antibodies is required, the eluate must be separated from the stain and titrated before the addition of indicator cells.

The Use of Low Ionic Strength Solution (LISS) as a Means of Improving the Efficiency of the Elution Technique

A recipe for a low ionic strength solution which facilitated antigen-antibody reaction without inducing detectable nonspecific uptake of antibody was introduced by Löw and Messeter.[9] Their main aim was to develop a method for increasing the rate of uptake of antibody by red cells as a basis for a quick, reliable compatibility test prior to blood transfusion. At a time when blood transfusion serologists were, understandably, still dabbling their toes in LISS, we had found that LISS so dramatically improved our tests for antigens in stains that we quickly introduced it for routine use.[11] The advantage for stain work is not the increase in the rate of reaction that LISS induces but its ability to increase the total amount of antibody taken up by an antigen, particularly if the long absorption time allowed for the uptake of anti-body by antigen in a stain is allowed. The suspension of the indicator cells in LISS for the detection of the eluted antibody is also an advantage. The effectiveness of LISS added both at absorption of antibody and for the detection of eluted antibody is shown in Fig 2 in which agglutination scores of the eluates with or without LISS are plotted against each other. Attention is particularly drawn to the number of stains in which no antigen at all would have been detectable without LISS. The results shown are for D and anti-D.

LISS benefits tests on older stains. Weak results obtained because of the age of the stain often become well defined. Table 9 shows repre-

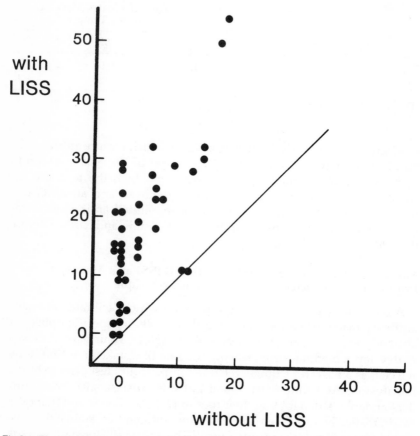

Fig 2.—The titration scores obtained with LISS used both at the absorption stage and for the titration of eluates compared with scores omitting LISS at both stages of the micro-elution technique performed on a series of bloodstains. (Data from McDowall et al.[11])

sentative stains of different ages tested for a variety of red cells antigens. It has been compiled to show not only the effect of LISS but to give an idea of the degree of agglutination that may be expected in bloodstain identification. It is of interest that while the reactions of anti-Fy^a are seen to be equally good with and without LISS, tests with anti-Fy^b are improved with LISS. The effect of LISS on Duffy antisera varies. In common with the experience of other workers, an anti-K susceptible to improvement by LISS has not been found. LISS does not benefit tests for the antigens of the ABO systems in stains.

Table 9.—Typing of Bloodstains for Various Antigens Showing Scope of Tests and Effect of LISS

Antiserum	Phenotype of Stain	Age in Weeks	Activity of Eluate from Stain	
			Without LISS	With LISS
Anti-C	Cc	3	±	+ + + +
Anti-E	Ee	28	±	+ +
Anti-Fy^a	Fy(a+b+)	20	+ + +	+ + +
Anti-Fy^b	Fy(a+b+)	20	±	+ +
Anti-Jk^a	Jk(a+b+)	32	—	+ + +
Anti-S	Ss	36	+ +	+ + + +

+ + + +, + + +, macroscopic agglutination
+ + good microscopic agglutination
± weak agglutination

Selection of Suitable Antisera for the Elution Technique

The ideal antibody for elution is one with a combining constant sufficiently high for efficient combination with the antigen but not so high that the antibody does not readily dissociate upon the application of heat. Such an antibody can be selected only by trial and error using stains of known type and various ages. The last requirement is important; antisera may be thoroughly satisfactory for typing fresh stains yet show a marked decrease in efficiency when tested against stains more than a few weeks old. The arrival of LISS has appreciably increased the number of suitable antisera. Antisera from which unwanted other antibodies have been removed or diluted out are preferable but it is not strictly necessary to eliminate contaminant antibodies so long as the chosen indicator cells do not react with them. It can never be taken for granted that antisera which are specific when used by other techniques will necessarily be specific when used for elution.

Monoclonal anti-A and anti-B reagents have been successfully used in our laboratory. There is a hint that certain anti-B monoclonal antibodies do not react with the B-like antigen produced by E coli and similar micro-organisms, the presence of which in stains can sometimes give rise to spurious positive reactions. If this is confirmed, it will increase the usefulness of monoclonal antibodies for stain work.

The Inhibition Test

Does the fact that a sensitive elution test has been developed for the detection of antigens in stains mean that there is now no place for the classical inhibition technique? For the detection of red cell antigens, the answer is yes. Although formerly M, N, Rh and K antigens were successfully detected in stains using the inhibition principle,[12-15] the amount of stained material required to show an unequivocal inhibition of the activity of the corresponding antibody is too large to make an inhibition test a practical procedure in most case work. For example, in a reported criminal case 2.5 sq cm of shredded cloth was used for the detection of the antigen K.[15]

A comparison between inhibition and elution techniques shown in Table 10 effectively demonstrates the superiority of elution for small amounts of antigen. Whereas there is no detectable inhibition of anti-s by either ss or Ss stains, when elution is performed on the actual material that was used in the inhibition test a strongly agglutinating anti-s is recovered in the eluates.

The inhibition test is, however, retained as an essential method for testing for A, B, H and Lewis substances in body fluid stains made

---

Table 10.—Comparison Between Inhibition and Elution Techniques Using Anti-s and 3 mm Sq Stains*

Ss	Type of Stain	Anti-s Titre Postinhibition	Elution Result
1)	Ss	4	+ + + + +
2)	SS	4	−
3)	ss	4	+ + + + +
4)	Ss	4	+ + + + +

*Data from Lincoln and Dodd.[16]

from saliva, seminal fluid, etc. Gm and Km types too are very success-fully demonstrated by inhibition.

For the detection of A, B and H soluble substances, the technique may be modified in three different ways according to the quantity and potency of the blood group substances present in the stain, which of course in case work is an unknown factor at the beginning of the investigation.

Method 1

Equal volumes of an extract from the stain in PBS and a suitably diluted antiserum (optimum titre 8-16) are mixed and after an incuba-tion period the mixture is titrated and its value compared with that of the original diluted antiserum.

Method 2

For increased sensitivity the antiserum is titrated and a volume of stain extract added to each dilution. This is compared with the original serum to which a volume of normal saline is added in place of the extract.

Method 3

If the antigen in the stain is very active, an extract is serially diluted and an equal volume of the antiserum added to each dilution followed, after incubation, with a volume of the appropriate red cells. At a certain dilution the antigen ceases to inhibit the antibody activity and agglutination appears.

It is an advantage to carry out the elution technique in parallel with inhibition as it is a sensitive technique for small quantities of group specific substances. Relied upon as the only technique, it has dis-advantages. It is sufficiently sensitive to detect the small amounts of A, B and H substances in nonsecretors and therefore does not offer a reliable indication of whether the stain originates from a secretor or nonsecretor. More important is the fact that when the concentration of antigen in the stain is very high no antibody is detectable in the eluate owing to antigen excess and a false negative test is obtained. In a recent case investigated in this laboratory, an extract of a seminal stain from a group O secretor which inhibited anti-H up to a dilution of the stain extract of 1 in 400 showed no sign whatever of anti-H in an eluate made from a thread of the stained material.

235

The Detection of HLA Antigens in Blood Stains

The HLA system is so richly polymorphic that it is an obvious target for research into the feasibility of identifying HLA antigen in blood stains. Lack of space necessitates brevity but since some of the most recent stain research has been in this field and has involved the inhibition principle it is relevant to include a summary of the work here.

Pamela Newall in Toronto and our team in London have between us attempted to type stains for a number of HLA antigens with some degree of success.[17, 18] Our results have shown that an inhibition technique based on inhibition of the lymphocyte toxicity reaction works well. Indeed, the inhibition of the activity of HLA antisera brought about by whole blood in the form of a stained thread is greater than that produced by a comparable suspension of fresh lymphocytes. The antigens too are fairly stable in older stains. The chief drawback is that a small number of false positives are obtained owing to the cross reactivities obtained with some antisera. These are unacceptable and will have to be overcome before HLA typing of stains is introduced into routine case work.

Summary

In spite of the loss of intact red cells through drying out when blood is shed and becomes a stain on clothing or hard surfaces, the antigens present remain detectable by special adaptation of techniques which make use of the principles of antigen-antibody reaction.

One of the most successful of these techniques is an elution procedure based on the well-known Landsteiner heat elution principle. To have become a worthwhile tool in everyday case work it has had to be adapted to detect the small amount of antigen present on a blood-stained thread of no more than 5 mm in length. The technique as modified for the detection of such small amounts of antigen and the correspondingly small amounts of antibody eluted therefrom, particularly with LISS incorporated in the tests, has proved so satisfactory that the detection of antigens in stains by the classical inhibition technique has been abandoned. The latter, however, has been retained as an essential method for the detection of A, B, H and Lewis substances in body fluid stains from seminal fluid, etc, and also for typing stains for Gm and Km markers.

Research in the field is pressing forward with encouraging attempts to detect HLA antigens in stains. These antigens seem to be surprisingly stable but there are some drawbacks owing to crossreactivity.

Appendix

A Microelution Technique for the Detection of Red Cell Antigens in Blood Stains

Bloodstained threads are attached to a polycarbonate sheet by means of a cellulose acetate glue composed of 1 part cellulose acetate to 2 parts acetone. It is convenient to mark out the sheet in small squares with a felt tip pen. Care must be taken to attach only the tip of each thread to the sheet to obtain the maximum length in contact with the antiserum.

A 3 mm length of thread is usually the optimum for ABH tests and 10 mm lengths for all other antigens.

Each antiserum, made up to half its selected dilution using AB serum, is added to an equal volume of LISS. For ABH tests the serum is diluted in PBS and the LISS is omitted.

Two drops of antiserum thus prepared are added to each stained thread and also to an appropriate unstained thread of the same material as a negative control. Bloodstained threads of known phenotype taken from stains of similar age to the test stains to provide a positive and negative control on each antiserum are included with each batch of tests.

The polycarbonate sheets are then placed in a well sealed moist chamber for incubation overnight at 4 C for ABH tests and 37 C for all other antigens.

After incubation excess serum is sucked off, the threads are then irrigated with ice cold saline after which the sheets are plunged in a tank of about 1 litre of saline at 4 C for two hours. During this period, the saline is changed once.

After washing, the threads are blotted dry and then cut off the sheet and transferred to separate tubes.

One generous drop of 0.3% bovine albumin in PBS is added and elution takes place in a shaking water bath for 15 minutes at 55 C for ABH, or 60 C for 30 minutes for Rh and other antigens.

Immediately at the end of the elution period one drop of indicator cells is added to each tube without removing the threads. These are at a concentration of 0.5% in 0.3% bovine albumin for ABH, 0.1% papain-treated cells in AB serum diluted 1 in 5 in LISS for Rh or for antigens requiring an AHG technique, the concentration is 1% in the AB serum/LISS diluent.

ABH tests are examined microscopically after 30 minutes at laboratory temperature on a rotatest machine followed by a final reading at two hours.

Rh tests are incubated for 1 hour at 37 C and then examined microscopically for agglutination. Additional sensitivity is sometimes gained by giving the tubes a short slow spin before reading.

Tests which require a final AHG technique (eg, Fy^a, Kell) are incubated at 37 C for 1 hour after which the threads and any supernatant fluid are removed, the cells are washed 3 times before adding AHG for a spin-AHG test, or the cells can be transferred to a drop of AHG reagent on a tile.

References

1. Lincoln PJ. Detection of antigens in stains. Proceedings of the 8th International Meeting of the Society of Forensic Haemogenetics. London 1979;153.
2. Lincoln PJ. Blood group evidence for the defence. Med Sci Law 1980;20:239.
3. Coombs RRA, Dodd BE. Possible application of the principle of mixed agglutination in the identification of blood stains. Med Sci Law 1961;1:359.
4. Coombs RRA, Bedford D, Rouillard LM. A and B blood group antigens or human epidermal cells demonstrated by mixed agglutination. Lancet 1956;1:461.
5. Kind SS. Absorption-elution grouping of dried bloodstains on fabrics. Nature 1960;187:789.
6. Nickolls LC, Pereira M. Modern methods of grouping dried bloodstains. Med Sci Law 1962;2:172.
7. Lincoln PJ, Dodd BE. The detection of the Rh antigens C, C^w, c, D, E, e and the antigen S of the MNSs system, in blood stains. Med Sci Law 1968;8:288.
8. Lincoln PJ, Dodd BE. An evaluation of the factors affecting the elution of antibodies from bloodstains. J Forens Sci Soc 1973;13:37.
9. Löw B, Messeter L. Antiglobulin test in low-ionic strength salt solution for rapid antibody screening and crossmatching. Vox Sang 1974;26:53.
10. Lincoln PJ, Dodd BE. The use of low ionic strength solution (LISS) in elution experiments and in combination with papain treated cells for the titration of various antibodies including eluted antibody. Vox Sang 1978;34:221.
11. McDowall MJ, Lincoln PJ, Dodd BE. Increased sensitivity of tests for the detection of blood group antigens in stains using a low ionic strength medium. Med Sci Law 1978;18:16.
12. Wiener AS. Blood groups and transfusion. 3rd ed. Springfield, IL: Charles C Thomas, chap 22.

13. Ducos J, Ruffié J. Recherches médico-légales des antigènes sanguins du type Rhésus dans les taches de sang sec. Acta Med Leg Soc 1954;3-4:111.
14. Ducos J. Absorption des anticorps anti-Kell par le sang desséché. Ann Med Leg 1957;37:1.
15. Jones AR, Diamond LK. Idenification of the Kell factor in dried bloodstains. J Forens Med 1955;2:243.
16. Lincoln PJ, Dodd BE. The application of a micro-elution technique using anti-human globulin for the detection of the S, s, K, Fy^a, Fy^b and Jk^a antigens in stains. Med Sci Law 1975;15:94.
17. Newall PJ, The identification of HLA-A2 and HLA-B5 antigens in dried bloodstains. J Can Soc Forens Sci 1979;12:1.
18. Hodge DG, Wolf E, Lincoln PJ, Festenstein H, Dodd BE. The detection of the HLA-A1 antigen in bloodstains. Med Sci Law 1980;20:213.

INDEX

A

Adsorption-Elution Tests, 194
  isolation, specific antibodies, 196
  multispecific sera, antibody identification, 195
  weak antigens and antibodies, detection, 194
Agglutination, History, 68
  lattice or crosslinking hypothesis, 68, 81
  Pollack's zeta potential theory, 69, 105
  surface charge and hydrophobicity, 68
  water and interfacial tension, 70
Agglutination, Latex Particle, 28, 33
  limitations, 33
Agglutination Potentiators, 99
  antibodies, complete and incomplete, 101
  bovine albumin, 103
  human serum and plasma, 102
  indirect antiglobulin reaction, 124
  practical uses, 113
  viscous solutions, 103
Agglutination, Red Blood Cell. *See* Red Blood Cell Agglutination.
Agglutination, Second Stage, 76
  albumin, 86
  attractive and repulsive forces, 76
  balance of forces, 80
  cationic polyelectrolytes, 88
  cholesterol, 90
  colloids, 87
  electrical double layer, 77
  hydration repulsion, 77
  ionic conditions, 83, 85, 86
  ionic strength, 77
  membrane flexibility/aldehyde fixation, 90
  organic solvents, surface tension, tabular display, 79
  proteolytic enzymes, 88
  salt effects, surface tension, 25C, tabular display, 78
  spiculation, 92
Agglutination, Spontaneous, 114, 126
Albumin. *See* Agglutination, Second Stage, 86.
Albumin Layering, 116, 120
Antibodies, Complete and Incomplete, 101
  methods to complete agglutination, 102
  two-stage hemagglutination, 101

Antibodies, Polyclonal vs Monoclonal, 15
  availability, 16
  limiting features, 16
  response to antigens, 15
  techniques, 16, 17
Antibodies, Unexpected, Macromolecular Additives, 121
  bovine albumin polymers, 122
Antibody Detection, Automated, 122
  macromolecules used, 122
Antibody Elution, Red Cells, 175
  adsorption-elution tests, 194
  elution applications, 196
  elution methods, procedures, Appendices 1-6, 210-213
  historical review, 175
  mechanisms, 177
  outcome influences, 182
  positive DAT, blood sample evaluation, 188
  selection of elution methods, 200
Antibody-Free Red Cells, 197. *See* Elution Applications.
  allohemagglutination, dissociation, 197
  DMSO technique, 199
  immune complexes with chloroquine diphosphate, dissociation, 198
  ZZAP technique, 199
Antibody Detection, Potentiators, 117
  albumin layering, 120
  antiglobulin test, 117
  bovine albumin method, 118, 119
  centrifugation, 118
  saline suspension, 119
  test procedures, early, 117
  variety of test procedures, tabular display, 120
Antibody Tests, Polycation Aggregation, 123
  LIP test, 123
Antibody Uptake, 47
  definitions, 48
  environmental factors, 58
  hemagglutination reaction, 47
  physicochemical basis, 50
  schematic representation of IgG molecule, 49
Antigen Denaturation, 143
  amino acid reaction sites, MN SGP, (Ss SGP) tabular display, 150 (151)
  enzyme modification, 143

241

Antigen Denaturation (continued)

human antigens, hydrolytic enzyme reaction, tabular display, 144-147
isolation techniques, 154
M/N and S/s sialoglycoproteins, diagram and legend, 149
neuraminidase, 153, 154, 155
Antigen Topography, 1 *See also* Red Cell Membrane.
Antigen-Antibody Binding, Physicochemical Basis, 50
antibody "affinity," 57
coulombic, ionic or electrostatic bonds, 54
hydrogen bonds, 54
hydrophobic effects, 55
intermolecular distance on van der Waals forces, diagram, 55
law of mass action, 56
London repulsive forces, 55
mean association constant K_0, 57
rates of association, dissociation, 56
schematic representation, 52
stereochemical complementarity, 51
van der Waals attractive forces, 54
Antigen-Antibody Reactions, 1
environmental factors, 58
hemagglutination demonstration, tabular display, 59
IgG subclasses, frequencies and isoelectric ranges, 59
ionic strength, 60
pH, 59
practical considerations, 62
temperature, 58
Antigen-antibody Reactions, Practical Considerations, 62
BSA (bovine serum albumin), 63
LISS (low-ionic strength solution), 62
polycations, 62
proteases, 63
Antigen-Antibody Reactions, Red Cells, 156
direct agglutination, enhanced, 158
enzyme enhancement, 156
hemagglutination, 156
IgG immunoglobulin, diagram, 157
size and distance, 158, 159
tabular display, 160
transferases, 160
Antigen Typing, Antisera Potentiation, 113
albumin replacement, 115
bovine albumin, 114
D antigen typing, 113
methods used, 113

polymers used, 114
spontaneous agglutination, 114, 126
Stratton's sandwich technique, 115
Antigenic Determinants, 7
blood group antigen sites per RBC, tabular display, 8
commonly used methods, 7
IgG anti-D binding vesicles, tabular display, 10
membrane aspects of blood group, tabular display, 7
membrane associations and properties, 11
membrane-bearing component, 10 (tabular display, 11)
orientation, 9
topological distribution, 9
Antigens, New, 140
cryptantigen T, diagram, 141
globoside components, 142
glycosphingolipids, diagram, 142
hydrolytic enzymes, tabular display, 140
I antigen, diagram, 142
Antigen Reaction, Indirect, 124
ionic strength, 124, 125
Attractive and Repulsive Forces, 76, 80 *See* Agglutination, Second Stage.
hydrogen bonding, 76
hydrophobic interactions, 68, 77
ionic forces, 76
increase in agglutinability, 81
relation to agglutination, 76, 80

B

Balance of Forces, Agglutination, 80. *See* Agglutination, Second Stage.
Blood Group Antigens, 1
membrane structure, 1
Blood Group Serology, 23, 39
immunoassays, improvement, 39, 40
immunoassays, potential applications, 39
immunoassays, use in blood banking, 40
Blood Stain Analysis, 223
distinguishing blood types, tabular display, 224
origin of stain, 224
problems encountered, 223
stains of different origins, tabular display, 225, 226
Blood Stain, Antigen Detection, 226
inhibition test, 234
LISS, elution technique, 231
micro-elution technique, 227, 237

mixed agglutination, 226
suitable antisera, elution technique, 233
Bovine Albumin, 103, 114, 117
conglutination, 104
current hypothesis of potentiation, 105, 114-121
explanations for promotion, 104
molecular size, 104
polymers, 122

C
Cationic Polyelectrolytes, 88. *See* Agglutination, Second Stage.
coacervation, 88
relation to agglutination, 89
Cell Surface Tension. *See* Water Structure as Basis.
Chemical Composition, Red Membrane, 3
Chloroform Elution, 177, 212
materials, method, 212
Chloroquine Dissociation of IgG, 177, 213
materials, method, note, 213, 214
Cholesterol, 5. *See* Agglutination, Second Stage.
erythrocyte membrane, 90
occurrence, 91
relation to agglutination, 91
Cold Acid Elution, 177, 210
materials and method, 210
Colloids. *See* Agglutination, Second Stage, 87.

D
Definitions, Antibody Uptake, 48
antibody-combining sites, 49
antibody populations, 50
antigenic determinants, 48
blood group antibodies, 48
blood group antigens, 48
cross reactivity, 50
Double Antibody Sandwich Method, 27, 29
modified method, 27, 29
Dynamic Flux of Cellular Membranes, Hydrophobic Effect. *See* Hydrophobic Effect and Dynamic Flux of Cellular Membranes.

E
Electrostatic Repulsion and Zeta Potential, 70, 74, 80, 93, 105
ELISA Method, Indirect, 29
Eluates, Routine Tests, 189. *See* Elution Studies, Blood Sample Evaluation, Positive DAT.

diagnostic studies, 190
neonatal blood samples, 189 all others, 190
Elution Applications, 196
antibody-free red cells, 197
forensic medicine, 200
lectin purification, 196
placental eluates, 199
Elution by Sonication, 177, 213
materials and method, 213
Elution of Alloantibodies, 201
comparative studies, tabular display, 203
early data, 201
independent investigators, 204
recent studies, 201
Elution of Antibody, History, 175
freeze-thaw technique, 176
heat technique, 175
modifications, 176, 177
Elution Mechanisms, 176
alteration of pH, 180
chaotropic ions, 180
chloroquine diphosphate, 181
freeze-thawing, 179
hapten addition, 179
heat, 178
organic solvents, 181
sonication, 180
ZZAP reagent, 181
Elution Methods, Selection, 200
comparative studies, 201, 205
conclusions, 208
elution techniques, 205
organic solvents, hazards, 201
preparation time, 200
Elution Procedures, Materials and Method, 210-213. (*See also* individual names.)
chloroform, 177, 212
chloroquine dissociation of IgG, 177, 213
cold acid, 177, 210
lui easy-freeze, 177, 211
sonication, 177, 213
xylene, 177, 211
Elution Procedures, Sensitivity, 187. *See* Elution Techniques, Factors Influencing Outcome.
comments, 205
concentration effect, 187
potentiation effect, 187
Elution Studies, Blood Sample Evaluation, Positive DAT, 188
interpretation of results, 192
pretransfusion samples, 191
routine tests, 189

Elution Studies, Pretransfusion Samples, 191
  alloantibody formation detection, 191
  positive DAT results, tabular display, 192
Elution Techniques, Factors Influencing Outcome, 182
  nonspecific attachment of immunoglobulins to RBC, 184
  sensitivity, 187
  technical considerations, 182
Elution Techniques, 205. *See* Elution Methods, Selection.
  comparative studies, tabular display, 206, 207
  eluate analysis, 208
  factors influencing outcome, 182
  selection of samples, 205
  summary tabular display, 209
Elution Test Results, 192
  alloantibodies mimicking autoantibodies, 193
  autoantibodies mimicking alloantibodies, 192
Energy Transfer, 28, 32, 33
Environmental Factors on Antigen-Antibody Reactions. *See* Antigen-Antibody Reactions, Environmental Factors.
Enzyme Action and Use, Immunohematology, 133
  definition, 133
  new applications, 162
  serological uses, 139
Enzyme Classification, Nomenclature, 134
  hydrolytic enzymes, classes and substrates, tabular display, 134
Enzyme, Criteria for Choosing, Tabular Display, 35
Enzyme Conjugates, 35 Tabular Displays:
  criteria for choosing enzyme, 35
  enzyme-antibody conjugation methods, 36
Enzyme Immunoassay, (EIA), 23, 25
  Chemical reactions, 42
Enzyme Multiplied Immunoassay Technique (EMIT), 28, 30
  formulae, 43
Enzyme Reaction Site Characteristics, 135
Enzyme Sources, 135
Enzyme-Antibody Conjugation Methods, Tabular Display, 36
Enzymes, Glycosidic, Immunochemical Studies, Tabular Display, 136
Enzymes, Hydrolytic, Serological Testing, Tabular Display, 138
Enzymes, New Applications, 162

ABH blood group system, 162
ELISA, 163
  IgG molecules, removal, 162
  McLeod syndrome screening, 163
Enzymes, Proteolytic, Immunohematology, Tabular Display, 137
Enzymes, Serological Uses, 139
  immunoglobulins, 161
  red cells, 139
  white cells and platelets, 160

F
Forensic Serology. *See* Serology, Forensic, 223.
Fluid Mosaic Model, RBC Membrane, 6
  mobility and interactions, 6

H
Haptens, 1, 30
  GIL haptens, 51
Hemagglutination, 1, 47
  phenomenon, 99
  pioneer investigations, 100
  tests, negative and positive, 99
Hemagglutination Reaction, 47
  coalescence stage, 47
  combination stage, 47
  relation to antibody uptake, 47
Histocompatibility to Complex in Man, 20
  relation to monoclonal antibodies, 20
HLA Antigen Detection, 236. *See* Serology, Forensic.
Hydrophobic Effect and Dynamic Flux of Cellular Membranes, 71
  agglutination effect, 72
  examples, 71

I
Immunoassay, Evolution, 24
  enzyme conjugates, 24
  homogeneous, 25
  immunofluorescent methods, 24
  radioimmunoassay, 24
Immunoassay, Fluorescence Excitation Transfer, 43
  methods, 43
Immunoassay, Fluorescent Polarization (FPIA), 28, 32
Immunoassay, Heterogeneous Enzyme (EIA), 25, 28-30
  differences from homogeneous assays, 30
Immunoassay, Homogeneous Enzyme, 30
  shortcomings, 30

Immunoassay, Homogeneous, Fluorescent, 38
Immunoassay, Nonisotopic, 23
  advantages, (tabular display) 23 (26)
  blood group serology, relation, 23, 39
  evolution of immunoassays, 24
  practical aspects, 34
  relation to other techniques, 23
  types, 25
Immunoassay, Practical Aspects, 34
  detection and automation, 39
  enzyme conjugates, 35
  fluorescent labels, 38
  solid phase, 29, 34, 35
  substrates, 37
Immunoassay, Spin, 28, 33
Immunoassay, Types, 25
  details of methods, 29-33
  EMIT advantages, 30
  environmental influences to fluorescent properties, 31
  recent developments, 30
Immunoassay, Types, Tabular Displays: 25, 26
  heterogeneous nonisotopic immunoassay, 27
  homogeneous/heterogeneous EIA with RIA and immunofluorescence, 26
  homogeneous nonisotopic immunoassay, 28
  nonisotopic immunoassay methods, 26
Immunoglobulins, Nonspecific Attachment to Red Cells, 184. See Elution Techniques, Factors Influencing Outcome.
  absence of preformed complex, 185
  cytophilic IgG, 185
  Matuhasi-Ogata phenomenon, 184
  significance, 186
Inhibition Test, 234. See Blood Stain, Antigen Detection.
  comparison of technique, different stains, tabular display, 234
  different methods, 235
Intramembranous Particles, 2
Ionic Conditions, Normal, 83. See also Agglutination, Second Stage.
  antigenic site density, 84
Ionic Strength, Antigen-Antibody Reactions, 60
  increased rate of association, 60
  increased uptake of antibody, 60
  increased uptake of complement, 62
  tabular display, 61
  theoretical considerations, 62

Ionic Strength, Decreased, 86. See Agglutination, Second Stage.
Ionic Strength, Increased, 85. See Agglutination, Second Stage.

L
Lipids, RBC Membrane, 5
  cholesterol, 5
  phospholipids, 5
  Rh antigen activity, 5
LISS, For Improving Elution Technique, 231
  blood stain typing, scope of tests, tabular display, 233
Lui Easy-Freeze Elution, 177, 211
  materials and method, 211

M
Macromolecules, 1, 10, 25
Membrane Structure, 1, 72
  chemical composition, RBC membrane, 3
  external domain, 73
  freeze-fracture techniques, 2
  intramembraneous particles, (IMP), 2
  lipids, 5, 72
  proteins, RBC membrane (tabular display), 2 (4)
  relation to blood group antigens, 1
  spectrin, 72
  ultrastructure, RBC membrane, 2
Micro-Elution Technique, 227. See Blood Stain, Antigen Detection.
  absorption stage, 228
  blood stains Anti-A:D at various temperatures, tabular display, 229
  decreasing amount of blood stain, antibody effect, tabular display, 228
  decreasing concentrations of anti-D, tabular display, 228
  detection of eluted antibody, 230
  different concentrations of cell suspension, titration of antibodies, tabular display, 230
  elution stage, 229
  papain, AHG technique, tabular display, 231
  red cell antigen detection, 237
Monoclonal Antibodies, 15
  major histocompatibility complex, 20
  membrane structure, 15
  parasites, 18
  polyclonal vs monoclonal, 15
  research implications, 20, 21
  tumor differentiation antigens, 19
  virus detection, 17

P

Parasites, Relation to Monoclonal Antibodies, 18
  detection of membrane structure, 18
Phospholipids, 5
Physicochemical Basis of Antigen-Antibody Binding. *See* Antigen-Antibody Binding, Physicochemical Reaction.
Potentiation, Human Serum or Plasma, 102
  conglutinin, 103
  relation to agglutination, 102
  slide test, 102
  test tube procedure, 103
Potentiation Hypotheses, 105
  enzyme treatment, experiment, 107
  ionic strength, 106
  synthetic polymers, 106
  water of hydration, 107
  zeta potential, 105
Potentiation Hypotheses, Alternative Suggestions, 108
  ferritin, clustering, 110
  heavy antigen density, 108
  morphology of red cell membrane, 112
  papain-treated and neuraminidase-treated cells, 109
  relevant antigen sites, 108
  spontaneous cellular aggregation, 111
  zeta potential, reduction, 110
Potentiators, Practical Uses, 113
  albumin layering, 116
  antibody detection, 117
  antigen typing, antisera, 113
  macromolecular additives, 121
  macromolecules in automated antibody detection, 122
  polycation aggregation in manual antibody tests, 123
Proteins, RBC Membrane, 3
  cytoskeleton, 5
  integral, 3
  major proteins, tabular display, 4
  peripheral, 3
  SDS-PAGE, 3, 4

R

Red Blood Cell Agglutination, 67
  definition, 67
  general concepts, 71
  history, 68
  second stage, agglutination, 76
Red Blood Cell, Electrostatic Repulsion and Zeta Potential, 74, 105. *See* Electrostatic Repulsion in Zeta Potential.

Red Blood Cells, Enzymes, 139
  antigen denaturation, 143
  enzyme modification, 139
  new antigens, 140
  proteolytic enzymes, 139
Red Blood Cell Membrane Structure, 72. *See* Membrane Structure.
Red Blood Cell, Water Structure and Interfacial Tension. *See* Water Structure as Basis for Cell Surface Interfacial Tension.
Red Cell Membrane, 1. *See also* Antigen Topography.
  antigenic determinants, 7
  blood group antigens and membrane structure, 1
  fluid mosaic model, 6

S

Serology, Forensic, 223. *See also* Blood Stain Analysis.
  antigen detection, blood stains, 226
  antigen-antibody techniques, 223
  HLA antigens, blood stains, 236
  microelution technique, 237
  problems, 224
  summary, 236
Spiculation, 92. *See* Agglutination, Second Stage.
  discocyte-echinocyte equilibrium, 92
Spin Immunoassay. *See* Immunoassay, Spin.
Stereochemical Complementarity, 51
  two-stage formulation of antigen-antibody complexes, 52
  variables of specific antigen:antibody complexes, tabular display, 53

T

T-Lymphocyte Subpopulation, 19, 21
Technical Considerations, Elution Techniques, 182. *See also* Elution Techniques, Factors Influencing Outcome.
  antibody dissociation, 183
  evaluation, 205
  improving efficiency, LISS, 231
  incomplete washing, 182
  incorrect technique, 183
  protein binding to glass surfaces, 183
  stability of eluates, 184
  storage changes, organic solvents, 183
Tumor Differentiation Antigens, 19
  human lymphocyte subpopulations, 19
  immunodeficiency states, 19, 20
  relation to monoclonal antigens, 19

V

Virus Detection, Monoclonal Antibodies, 17
    evolution of monoclonal antibodies, 18
    MCMV, 17
    methods, 17
    polyclonal antibody detection, 18

W

Water Structure as Basis for Cell Surface Interfacial Tension, 70, 73, 74, 80, 82, 93

White Blood Cells and Platelets, 160
    glycosyltransferases, immunohematology, tabular display, 161
    immunoglobulins, 161

X

Xylene Elution, 177, 211
    materials, methods, notes, 211-212